Acute Paediatric Pain Management

A Practical Guide

◆

edited by

NEIL S MORTON,
Consultant in Paediatric Anaesthesia,
Intensive Care and Pain Management,
Department of Anaesthesia,
Royal Hospital for Sick Children,
Glasgow
Senior Lecturer in Paediatric Anaesthesia
University of Glasgow

W.B. Saunders
London • Edinburgh • New York • Philadelphia
Sydney • Toronto

WB Saunders is an imprint of Harcourt Brace and Company Ltd

Harcourt Brace and
Company Ltd

24–28 Oval Road
London NW1 7DX

The Curtis Center
Independence Square West
Philadelphia, PA 19106–3399,
USA

Harcourt Brace & Company
55 Horner Avenue
Toronto, Ontario M8Z 4X6,
Canada

Harcourt Brace & Company,
Australia
30–52 Smidmore Street
Marrickville, NSW 2204,
Australia

A catalogue record for this book is available from the British
Library

ISBN 0–7020–2219–5

Typeset by J&L Composition Ltd, Filey, North Yorkshire
Printed and bound in Great Britain by WBC Book
Manufacturers Ltd, Bridgend, Mid Glamorgan

CONTENTS

Ms Susan Fisher
Clinical Nurse Specialist in Pain Relief
Royal Hospital for Sick Children
Yorkhill NHS Trust
Glasgow
Scotland, UK

Dr Tom G. Hansen
Consultant Paediatric Anaesthetist
Department of Anaesthesia and Intensive Care Medicine
Odense University Hospital
Denmark

Dr Steen W. Henneberg
Consultant Paediatric Anaesthetist
Department of Anaesthesia
Juliane Marie Centret
Rigshospitalet
Denmark

Dr G.A.M. Wilson
Specialist Registrar
Department of Anaesthesia
Royal Hospital for Sick Children
Edinburgh
Scotland, UK

Dr Ros A. Lawson
Consultant Paediatric Anaesthetist
Department of Anaesthesia
Royal Hospital for Sick Children
Yorkhill NHS Trust
Glasgow
Scotland, UK
formerly Staff Anaesthetist
Seattle Childrens' Hospital
Seattle, USA

Dr Kay O'Brien
Specialist Senior Registrar in Paediatric Anaesthesia
Department of Anaesthesia
Royal Hospital for Sick Children
Yorkhill NHS Trust
Glasgow
Scotland, UK

Dr Eddie Doyle
Consultant Paediatric Anaesthetist
Department of Anaesthesia
Royal Hospital for Sick Children
Edinburgh
Scotland, UK

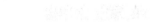

T he aim of this book is to provide a paediatric text to compliment the excellent book from W.B. Saunders by Pam McIntyre and Brian Ready *Acute Pain Management – A Practical Guide*. There has been a huge increase in interest in paediatric pain management in the last 10 years but despite the evidence base for good practice, many children suffer unnecessary pain for want of simple measures. I have tried to point out the important differences between children and adults in pain physiology, assessment, pharmacology and treatment. It is a practical guide and has to be didactic but I have tried to give a choice of techniques to cope with nearly all acute pain situations in children. Examples of protocols, guidelines, information leaflets and monitoring charts are included for illustrative purposes and can be adapted to local needs. Controversial areas are discussed and mentioned and solutions presented where possible and a series of acute pain management plans is given for those who like the recipe book approach! Sedation of children for procedures is discussed in detail as this is a field where standards often slip. I hope the readers of this book will find practical help and guidance on prevention and management of acute pain in children. The challenge for all of us is to ensure that these techniques are made available to *all* children who need them, not just the fortunate few.

N.S. Morton
Glasgow
1998

ACKNOWLEDGEMENTS

I would like to express my sincere thanks to all the contributors to this book and to the publishers and their expert assessors for their helpful comments. In particular, I wish to thank all those involved with the pain management service at the Royal Hospital for Sick Children in Glasgow and my senior colleagues for their support. The care of children has hilarious, happy, poignant and sad moments but is always rewarding.

N.S. Morton
Glasgow
1998

AAG	alpha-l-acid glycoprotein
ACTH	adrenocorticotrophic hormone
a & e	accident & emergency
APRS	acute pain relief service
bd	twice daily
BP	blood pressure
bpm	beats per minute
c/i	contraindications
CNS	central nervous system
CRF	corticotrophin releasing factor
CRPS	complex regional pain syndrome
CSF	cerebrospinal fluid
EMLA	eutectic mixture of local anaesthetics
ENT	ear, nose and throat
GFR	glomerular filtration rate
GI	gastrointestinal
HbA	adult haemoglobin
HbF	foetal haemoglobin
HDU	high dependency unit
HR	heart rate
ICU	Intensive Care Unit
im, IM	intramuscular
ITU	Intensive Therapy Unit
iv, IV	intravenous
IVM	intravenous morphine
IVPCAM	intravenous patient controlled analgesia with morphine
m	month
NABQI	N-acetyl-p-benzoquinoneimine
NCA	Nurse-controlled analgesia
NMDA	N-methyl D-aspartate
NSAID	non-steroidal anti-inflammatory drugs
o/pr	orally/rectally
pca, PCA	patient controlled analgesia
PICU	Paediatric Intensive Care Unit

PONV	postoperative nausea and vomiting
pr	per rectum (rectally)
prn	pro re nata (as required)
RHSC	Royal Hospital for Sick Children, Glasgow
RR	respiratory rate
sc, SC	subcutaneous
SCM	subcutaneous morphine infusion
SCPCAM	subcutaneous patient controlled analgesia with morphine
SpO_2	oxygen saturation by pulse oximetry
TENS	transcutaneous electrical nerve stimulation
UDP	uridine diphosphate
VT	ventricular tachycardia
y	year

Important notice

Every effort has been made to check the drug dosages given in this book. However, as it is possible that dosage schedules have been revised, the reader is strongly urged to consult the drug companies' literature before administering any of the drugs listed.

CHAPTER 1

PAIN PREVENTION AND MANAGEMENT IN CHILDREN

Susan Fisher, Neil S. Morton

Principles

Education

Planning pain management

PRINCIPLES

Pain is defined by the International Association for the Study of Pain as 'an unpleasant sensory and emotional experience associated with actual or potential tissue damage or described in terms of such damage'. There are long term psychological and physical consequences of inadequate pain control in all age groups (**Box 1.1**).

It is now accepted that for moral, humanitarian, ethical and physiological reasons, pain should be anticipated and safely and effectively controlled in all children, whatever their age, maturity or severity of illness (**Box 1.2**).

Techniques of pain control should be applied in advance of the painful stimulus wherever possible. This pre-emptive approach helps to minimize the emotional problems of fear and anxiety, prevents the 'wind-up' phenomenon of central nervous system sensitization to

---

Risks of untreated pain

Psychological
- anxiety and fear (now and in the future)
- nightmares and sleep disturbance
- behavioural and personality disturbance
- disruption of schooling
- development of vicious cycles to chronic pain

Physical
- increased death rate after major surgery
- increased morbidity

    respiratory: hypoxaemia, impaired respiratory function, decreased cough and cooperation with physiotherapy, increased secretion retention, atelectasis, infection

    cardiovascular: sympathetic stimulation (increased heart rate and blood pressure, vasoconstriction, altered regional blood flow, increased oxygen consumption), risk of venous thrombosis

    stress response: stress hormone surges, disordered electrolyte and fluid balance, high blood sugar level, osmotic diuresis in neonates, depressed immune function

    cerebral: increase in intracranial pressure, increased risk of intraventricular haemorrhage or cerebral ischaemia in premature neonates

    musculoskeletal: muscle spasms, immobility, delayed mobilisation

    visceral: slowing of gastrointestinal and urinary function

    wound: decreased healing

Box 1.1

noxious stimuli and tissue release of pain mediators, ameliorates the stress response and reduces the intra-operative anaesthetic requirement and subsequent analgesic requirements. A multimodal approach to preventing pain using local anaesthetics, opioids, non-steroidal anti-inflammatory drugs (NSAIDs), sedation and non-drug methods in a safe and effective planned way, tailored to each individual child's needs, is the basis of acute pain prevention. This requires that pain is

---

▼ **Benefits of pain prevention and control**

- humanitarian
- moral and ethical
- psychological: patient satisfaction, reduced anxiety and fear, normalized sleep and behaviour, avoidance of vicious cycles to chronic pain
- physical: lower mortality after major surgery, decreased cardiorespiratory complications, earlier weaning from respiratory support, decreased wound and respiratory infection rates, earlier mobilization and discharge, earlier return of visceral function and oral intake, better fluid and electrolyte homeostasis, reduced cerebral complications

Box 1.2

▼ **Risks of pain control**

- technique: needle damage, needle misplacement, haematoma, cerebrospinal fluid leak, infection, urinary retention, itch, extravasation of drug, depot effect with subcutaneous/intramuscular route
- drug: allergy, overdose, underdose, prescription error, dilution error, wrong drug, adverse effect
- infusion equipment: over-infusion, under-infusion, gravity free-flow, reflux, electronic interference, extravasation

Box 1.3

assessed regularly and the assessment is linked to action to maintain pain control with minimal adverse effects (**Box 1.3**).

Preparing the child and family in advance with good written and verbal information and careful matching of the analgesic technique to the child will help to reduce fear and anxiety and correct misconceptions. This approach should apply to all painful procedures however minor or major, and often means placing pain prevention higher up the list of priorities in each child's overall plan of care. This requires good education of staff, parents and children, forward planning and organization. A paediatric pain management service has been found to be effective in achieving consistent standards of efficacy and safety (**Box 1.4**).

EDUCATION

Studies have shown that one of the major reasons for poor paediatric pain management is a lack of education of staff, parents and children. Myths and misconceptions persist, for example that children do not feel pain

---

Roles of a paediatric pain management service

- organization: personnel, 24–hour cover, call-out and consultation system, good communication systems, equipment, teaching, clinic for complex/long term cases
- service delivery: multidisciplinary personnel (pain nurse, specialist, anaesthetist, pharmacist, physiotherapist, paediatrician, surgeon, psychologist, psychiatrist, play therapist, etc.), monitoring standard, equipment, follow-up system, daily senior anaesthetic input
- education: programme for anaesthetists, surgeons, paediatricians, emergency room staff, nurses, pharmacists, parents, children, management personnel
- audit: efficacy, safety, adverse events, outcome, equipment, costs, efficiency
- research: drugs, equipment, monitoring, benefits, risks

Box 1.4

as much as adults or are at risk of addiction if opioids are used. Many medical staff are still worried about the safety aspects of prescribing adequate doses of analgesia for children. Medical and nursing students and trainees have often received very little formal training in paediatric pain management but are expected to prescribe and administer analgesia to children. As a result, staff often express undue concern about side effects and tend to use inadequate doses of analgesic drugs. Many nurses are trained to await the patient's demand for analgesia and are not familiar with pre-empting pain and the concept of giving concurrent analgesics with different modes of action, i.e. multimodal pain control or balanced analgesia, with comments such as 'this child is already getting morphine, he doesn't need an NSAID or paracetamol too'. Fears regarding opioid addiction often lead to a premature change to a weaker analgesic. Medical and nursing staff tend to underestimate pain in children and this is borne out by studies of the assessments of pain made by children themselves when compared to the assessments made by parents or staff. Many staff still feel that pain can only be reduced but not controlled or prevented.

Practice can be changed by education. This is illustrated by the changes in perception and practice amongst paediatric anaesthetists surveyed in 1988 and again in 1995 (**Table 1.1**). This highlights very well the evolution of more comprehensive analgesic prescribing and more appropriate use of local anaesthetics, opioids and NSAIDs.

MEDICAL STAFF
Medical staff may be taught about pain theories and may be aware of the anatomy and physiology of pain but are often not aware of the practical aspects. They need to

Table 1.1 Results of two surveys of paediatric anaesthetists' perceptions and practice in 1995 compared with 1988 (de Lima et al., 1996)

	1988	1995
% who thought neonates did not feel pain	13%	0%
% who prescribed opioids for neonates after major surgery	10%	91%
% who used local anaesthetic block or infiltration in newborns	27%	88%
% who used local anaesthetic for minor surgery	27%	99%

know how to assess paediatric pain efficiently and learn how to intervene effectively with both drug and non-drug methods. The range of analgesic techniques, drugs and their doses, interactions and adverse effects should be taught.

NURSING STAFF

The nurse at the bedside is often the first line of safety for the patient. It is vital that nurses are aware of drug effects, doses, interactions and possible side effects. They must learn to assess pain in children regularly and to link these assessments to action using a range of analgesic techniques, both simple and complex, pharmacological and non-pharmacological. Recognition and management of adverse effects must be clearly taught for each technique. A flexible approach based upon regular reassessment of pain and titration of analgesia works best and it is well recognized that ward routines, set times for drug rounds and shortage of staff cause problems in delivering effective and safe analgesia for all children to a consistent standard.

Organization of educational opportunities can be difficult in busy wards. Bedside teaching with one-to-one explanations is very effective and enhances two-way communication between the surgical team and the pain team, which is extremely important. Workshops, tutorials, lectures, written information and practical assessment on the ward are all helpful (**Box 1.5**).

PARENT AND PATIENT EDUCATION

Information should be provided in an appropriate language and in written and verbal forms. Parents may ask about the drugs their child may receive and should be given detailed explanations about the options available. The benefits and risks should be clearly explained. If the child is old enough to be consulted then they can be asked about their preferences and should receive an explanation in a form relevant to their age and development. Information booklets again can be very useful. Information may need to be repeated several times depending on the circumstances. For example, the young or very ill child may not be able to understand instructions, and parents may be too upset to absorb information. In these

---

Priorities of nurse education

- principles of multimodal analgesia
- pain assessment in children
- monitoring techniques
- infusion device safety
- analgesic drugs, doses, indications, contraindications and potential adverse effects
- detection and management of adverse effects
- non-drug methods of pain management
- liaison with other disciplines

Box 1.5

circumstances, printed information is useful in reinforcing verbal explanations and can be given out to parents and patients for later reference (see **Appendices 3, 5 and 7**).

A specific plan of analgesia can then be tailored to the needs of each individual child. If parents are familiar with a particular technique such as patient-controlled analgesia, they can encourage their children to use the technique more appropriately. Clear information should help to decrease the level of anxiety and in turn this reduces the analgesic requirement. Parents can also help with assessment of their child, particularly when the child has a mental handicap or has behavioural or developmental problems. The parent is often best at distinguishing the signs of pain in their child and should be encouraged to communicate with staff so that effective analgesia can be maintained. Although a high proportion of parents are resident with their child in hospital, they are more likely to be confident about leaving their child in the care of others if the child is comfortable. A family centred approach to the care of children is very helpful in encouraging the child back towards their normal environment and level of function.

EDUCATION OF OTHER STAFF

A multidisciplinary approach to pain management is essential and liaison between anaesthetists, nurses, surgeons, paediatricians, physiotherapists, play therapists, psychologists and psychiatrists will be needed to optimize care of individual children. The pain management service can act as coordinator of these various disciplines and provides a valuable education resource for these specialities. Accreditation and re-accreditation schemes for both knowledge and competence are to be recommended (**Box 1.6**).

Training targets

- children: information in a form appropriate to the level of understanding, aware of available techniques, risks and benefits, what to expect, what should work for them, how to cope, pain management service, side effects and treatment available, pain assessment methods, limitations of techniques, how to call for help if analgesia is inadequate or side effects are too severe, special tuition for PCA
- parents: above in more detail, monitoring for adverse effects, risks of addiction, importance of calling early for help
- ward nurse: analgesic techniques, monitoring standards, pain assessment techniques, troubleshooting, recognition and management of adverse effects, infusion device training and safety, administration of rescue analgesia, when to call for help, paediatric and neonatal basic life support, preparing opioid infusion syringes
- high dependency or intensive care nurse: above plus advanced paediatric and neonatal life support techniques and drugs, extended role in intravenous opioid administration and epidural management and monitoring, programming PCA devices
- specialist pain nurse: above plus teaching, audit and research, design and operation of protocols, drug interactions, transcribing simple analgesic prescriptions, consultations, chronic pain assessment and management, procedural pain management
- trainee medical staff: above plus prescribing within protocols, extra training if working in HDU and ICU
- trainee anaesthetic staff: above plus detailed aspects of conduct of local and regional analgesia, epidural management, safe sedation of children
- consultant medical staff: above plus knowledge of the range of available techniques and their indications and contraindications (c/I), when to ask for a pain consultation
- consultant anaesthetic staff: above plus selection and implementation of appropriate pain prevention and management plans, design of protocols

Box 1.6

▼ ## Factors in planning pain management

- age, maturity, physical status, mental status
- severity of illness
- medical factors: e.g. organ dysfunction, asthma, epilepsy, reflux
- surgical factors: e.g. extent and nature of surgery
- anaesthetic factors: e.g. airway abnormality, suitability or c/i to particular analgesic technique
- expected pain severity and duration
- pain assessment method and training of assessor
- past pain experience
- child/parental preferences
- psychological factors
- medical environment: day case, outpatient, a & e, general ward, HDU, ITU
- can minimum monitoring standard be met: nurse dependency, assessment of efficacy, monitoring and management of adverse effects, infusion device safety
- anticipated pathway to recovery
- continuing pain control

Box 1.7

PLANNING PAIN MANAGEMENT

There are many factors to consider when planning individualized pain management (**Box 1.7**).

Pain management plans for specific patient groups are detailed in Chapter 10.

KEY LEARNING POINTS

- prevention of pain and good pain control are high priorities when dealing with children
- the benefits of pain control techniques, when properly selected and applied, outweigh the risks

- education of children, parents and staff improves the success and safety of pain control
- to ensure *comprehensive* pain prevention and control requires planning and organization

REFERENCE AND FURTHER READING

de Lima J., Lloyd-Thomas A.R., Howard R.F., Sumner E. and Quinn T.M. (1996) Infant and neonatal pain: anaesthetists' perceptions and prescribing patterns. *British Medical Journal* **313**, 787.

Derbyshire S.W.G., Furedi A., Glover V., Fisk N., Szawarski Z., Lloyd-Thomas A.R. and Fitzgerald M. (1996) Do foetuses feel pain? *British Medical Journal* **313**, 795–799.

Howard R.F. (1996) Planning for pain relief. *Bailliere's Clinical Anaesthesiology* **10**, 657–675.

McIntyre P.E. and Ready L.B. (1996) *Acute Pain Management: A Practical Guide*. WB Saunders, London.

McQuay H., Moore A. and Justins D. (1997) Treating acute pain in hospital. *British Medical Journal* **314**, 1531–1535.

Notcutt W.G. (1997) What makes acute pain chronic? *Current Anaesthesia and Critical Care* **8**, 55–61.

Ready L.B. and Edwards W.T. (1992) *Management of Acute Pain: A Practical Guide*. IASP Publications, Seattle.

Royal College of Paediatrics and Child Health (1997) *Prevention and Control of Pain in Children*. BMJ Publishing Group, London.

Walco G.A., Cassidy R.C. and Schechter N.L. (1994) Pain, hurt, and harm. The ethics of pain control in infants and children. *New England Journal of Medicine* **331**, 541–544.

CHAPTER 2

DEVELOPMENT OF PAEDIATRIC PAIN PERCEPTION

Neil S. Morton

Overview of pain mechanisms
Development of pain mechanisms in the
peripheral tissues
Development of pain mechanisms in the
central nervous system
Development of the endocrine and
metabolic stress response
Long term consequences of neonatal pain or
exposure to analgesics
Development of the brain and emotional responses

OVERVIEW OF PAIN MECHANISMS

The pain process is complex and involves physical, chemical and emotional components. The effective management of pain must deal with each of these components in an integrated way with physical, pharmacological and psychological aspects of treatment. **Figure 2.1** represents tissue damage directly activating pain nerves or sensitizing the pain nerve so that it is more easily activated. This latter process is a positive feedback loop which is often called 'wind-up' and means that smaller, even non-noxious stimuli will produce

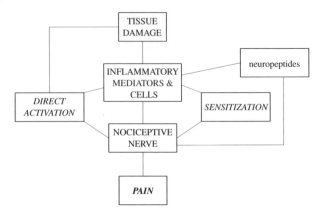

Figure 2.1
Overview of pain mechanisms

activation of the pain nerves. The physical stimulus producing pain must be converted or *transduced* into an electrical impulse (action potential) which involves movement of charged chemicals (ions) through ion channels in nerves. This happens at special nerve endings (nociceptors) throughout the body tissues which convert the energy of the physical stimulus into action potentials. These are then *transmitted* along a series of nerves (Aδ and C fibres) and across nerve junctions (synapses). At each junction and in several complex ways the transmission of the nerve impulses can be modified or *modulated* to increase or decrease onward transmission to the central nervous system (i.e. the spinal cord and brain). Within the central nervous system, modulation also occurs and finally the sensation is perceived at the level of the cerebral cortex (**Figure 2.2**).

Links with other parts of the brain result in emotional and behavioural effects of the unpleasant signals which are shown in different ways at different

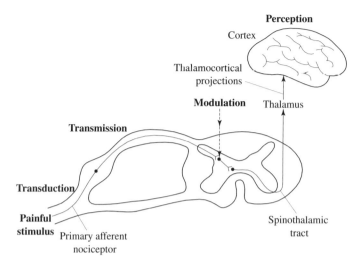

Figure 2.2
The pain pathway

stages of development but include crying, expression
on the face, body positioning, withdrawal and limitation
of mobility and function.

The pain pathway therefore leads from nociceptors in
the tissues via the primary afferent input nerves to the
dorsal horn of the spinal cord and onwards up the tracts
leading from the spinal cord to the lower centres of the
brain and projecting from there to higher centres in the
cortex. From the brain descending control signals are
sent to modulate the signals coming into the spinal cord.
The autonomic nervous system conducts noxious
signals into the central nervous system from the visceral
tissues but also sends signals out to the spinal cord to
modulate the input from tissue nociceptors to the
central nervous system. The idea of modulation of
noxious stimuli in the spinal cord has been called the
gate control theory. The gate is opened to allow stimuli

to reach the brain by a flood of stimuli conducted by small diameter pain fibres and closed by stimuli conducted by large diameter fibres and descending inhibitory signals from the brain. A good analogy is to think of the spinal cord as a computer chip with many on and off switches and the proportions of these determine how much stimulation is transmitted on up to the brain to be perceived. An excessive or prolonged painful input may have long lasting effects and this may include changes in the structure of the 'chip' which make it ultra-sensitive to painful inputs. This then can be the start of the vicious cycles which may cause pain to persist and become chronic (Notcutt, 1997).

DEVELOPMENT OF PAIN MECHANISMS IN THE PERIPHERAL TISSUES

Although there are sensory nerve endings in neonatal skin, these are not located or organized in the same way as in the adult. The response of the tissues to injury or wounding is different in the newborn. The combination of these factors markedly affects the responses of the newborn to tissue damage.

INNERVATION OF THE SKIN

There are sensory nerve terminals in the skin from around 7 weeks which have spread to all body surfaces by 22–29 weeks of gestation. These are in the form of plexuses located in the dermis and the epidermis. Over time in the neonate these plexuses become more complicated and more deeply situated in the dermis. This corresponds with hair follicles appearing and becoming innervated by myelin coated nerves. Small branches with no myelin sheaths grow out into the epidermis. Sympathetic nerves are deeply situated at birth below the dermis but grow into the dermis to supply blood vessels and hair follicle structures such as the piloerector muscles. The growth of all these nerves is probably controlled by the local concentration of nerve growth factor. The overall effect of growth of nerve terminals into the surface layers of the skin is that the sensory threshold stays roughly the same over development despite the increasing thickness of the skin as the infant grows. However, because the organization is immature both in the periphery and centrally, with large terminal fields for sensory neurones, the responses produced by skin stimuli are not very specific, have a low threshold for producing a response and are not very precisely localized in space.

INFLAMMATORY RESPONSE IN TISSUES

It is well known that foetal wounds heal incredibly quickly with hardly any scarring. This is due to differences in the immune system in the foetus and newborn who repair wounds using macrophages rather than polymorphs. This is because the numbers of polymorphs are small and their functions are poorly developed (less movement to chemical stimuli, less ingestion of solid particles and less bacterial killing capacity). The tissue macrophages release many types of chemical which stimulate cell growth, cell division, nerve growth and the attraction of other cells into the local area to secrete their local hormones. The effect of this macrophage-based process is rapid, scar-free healing with extra local nerve growth.

SPROUTING OF NERVE TERMINALS IN WOUNDED SKIN

In neonates, wounding of the skin results in massive sprouting of the sensory nerve endings in and near the wound. This response is much more marked than in the adult. This produces a state of hyperinnervation of the wounded area for many weeks after the wound has healed. This wounded region has a lowered threshold for sensations and can thus be said to be hypersensitive to all kinds of stimuli. The later in development that the wound occurs, the less sprouting is seen. This is because, in the neonate, both larger myelinated A fibres and smaller unmyelinated C fibres are involved in the sprouting response, whereas in adults only C fibres sprout. The vigorous sprouting response in the neonate is probably due to the release of nerve growth factors. The reason for sprouting may be to increase the transport to the wound via the nerve endings of peptides involved in healing. However, the fact that wounds in the neonatal period become oversupplied with sensory nerve endings and are hypersensitive for many weeks after the wound has healed is very important clinically. What is not yet known is whether locally applied or systemic analgesics affect this sprouting response and indeed if it is desirable to prevent sprouting if it is involved in healing.

SPROUTING OF NERVES IN THE SPINAL CORD IN RESPONSE TO PERIPHERAL NERVE DAMAGE

A similar nerve sprouting response can occur in the spinal cord after peripheral nerve damage and this can alter the sensory map thereafter. This means that peripheral stimuli will produce more widespread and extensive effects on the central nervous system.

DEVELOPMENT OF PAIN MECHANISMS IN THE CENTRAL NERVOUS SYSTEM

ORGANIZATION OF PAIN PATHWAYS

The larger A fibres from the skin enter the dorsal horn of the spinal cord quite early in development and extend to many of the layers of the dorsal horn for a period lasting several weeks. They also extend into the area known as the substantia gelatinosa in the spinal cord. Smaller unmyelinated C fibres also grow into this area some time after the A fibres and so for a few weeks the A and C fibre territories overlap. Later, the A fibres become more restricted to the deeper layers of the dorsal horn. The substantia gelatinosa takes a long time to mature and C fibres become wired up to the cells in this area over many weeks (**Figure 2.3**). The effects of this overlap of nerve terminals is that even small, non-noxious stimuli can produce large, non-selective responses that are not very precisely organized in time and space and these are indistinguishable from the effects of noxious stimuli.

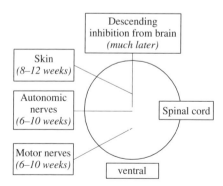

Figure 2.3
Timing of the development of connections from the peripheral nervous system into the spinal cord

Thus the neonatal response to almost any sensory stimulus will be low threshold, non-specific and poorly organized. This means that to assess and interpret the responses is very difficult as the responses to so many stimuli are alike. The sick, premature or critically ill baby's responses tend to be obtunded and even less specific. This is why measurement of pain in the neonate, particularly when they are ill, is so difficult.

EXCITATORY SYSTEMS

The main excitatory pain systems in the central nervous system are (1) glutamate acting on NMDA receptors and (2) neuropeptides acting on neurokinin receptors (e.g. Substance P). The receptors for these excitatory systems are much more numerous and more widely distributed in the neonatal central nervous system and regress towards their adult locations over several weeks. This applies particularly to Substance P and the glutamate–NMDA systems. The structure and function of these receptors also differ in neonates and adults and the receptors undergo changes during development. For example, neonatal NMDA receptors are more sensitive to glutamate (**Box 2.1**).

Genetic changes also occur in the spinal cord in response to sensory stimulation. In the newborn, innocuous stimuli can activate these gene switches, whereas in adults painful stimuli are needed. Thus in the neonatal central nervous system there are more excitatory receptors, distributed more widely and more easily activated by their excitatory transmitters. The neonatal central nervous system is thus in a 'hyperexcitable' state. This is further accentuated by the underdevelopment of the inhibitory systems noted next.

▼

Chemicals involved in pain transmission	
Excitatory chemicals	*Inhibitory chemicals*
Substance P	somatostatin
neurokinin A	cholecystokinin
calcitonin gene-related peptide	galanin
NMDA	adenosine
AMPA	alpha-2–agonists
glutamate	

Box 2.1

INHIBITORY SYSTEMS

The neonate has a poorly developed system for inhibiting excitatory stimuli in the central nervous system and this contributes to the exaggerated responses to even innocuous stimuli. These inhibitory systems are of three main types and all develop after birth. Firstly, the C fibres entering into the substantia gelatinosa of the spinal cord trigger the maturation of interconnecting neurones which have important inhibitory functions. These local inhibitory neurones do not reach their targets for some time even though their receptor systems may be present. A good example to consider is the opioid receptor system. Mu, kappa and delta opioid receptors are present in early development. Their numbers increase in the early neonatal period and they are responsive to exogenously administered morphine. Morphine is more potent in early life when given systemically or when applied locally near the spinal cord. The neurones on which these receptors lie are not connected up till later in development and so stimulation of these nerves does not result in opioid receptor activation. Secondly, the descending inhibitory nerves growing down from the brainstem into the spinal cord do not send branches into the dorsal horn for some weeks after birth. Thirdly, neurotransmitters which in adults cause inhibition, may act as excitatory compounds in the immature nervous system (e.g. GABA, glycine). The overall effect is lack of inhibition in an already hyperexcitable system.

DEVELOPMENT OF THE ENDOCRINE AND METABOLIC STRESS RESPONSE

FOETAL PAIN AND STRESS

It is now well established that foetuses and neonates can mount a stress response from around 20 weeks gestation. Whether the foetus can feel pain is best considered in relation to the development of consciousness which requires organized brain activity. This probably develops as the cerebral cortex develops and becomes connected up. This might be thought of like a dimmer switch coming on gradually as the brain grows and matures. The full complement of 1000 million neurones is present by 20 weeks gestation and some EEG activity is seen from this time. Temporary connections reach the cortex from lower centres in the thalamus between 17 and 25 weeks and become permanent between 26 and 34 weeks. Evoked potentials start to become more complex between 29 and 40 weeks but are very slow and simple before 29 weeks.

The foetal stress response is mainly mediated by cortisol and catecholamines. The hypothalamus and pituitary become a functional unit from 21 weeks gestation and corticotrophin releasing factor (CRF) from the hypothalamus can cause release of ACTH and beta-endorphin from foetal tissues from 20 weeks onwards.

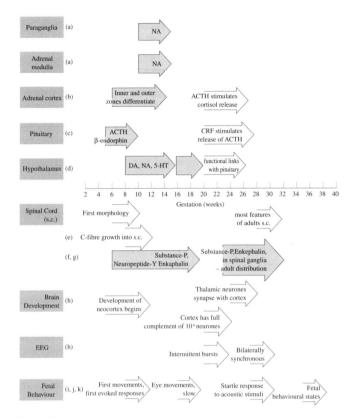

Figure 2.4
Foetal development; from Glover and Giannakoulpoulos (1995)
(copyright permission granted)

In the foetus, the adrenal cortex is 10–20 times the adult size in relation to body weight but shrinks by half in the first month of life. The foetus produces large amounts of steroid hormones but these are in different proportions to the neonate or child, with relatively little cortisol. The chromaffin tissues of the adrenal medulla and in the ganglia around the aorta contain noradrenaline from about 10 weeks gestation and release large amounts in

23

response to stress (e.g. in asphyxia). Adrenaline is also present beyond 23 weeks but in smaller amounts. A cortisol and beta-endorphin increase in response to intrauterine needling for exchange transfusion has been clearly shown in human foetuses as young as 23 weeks gestation. The implications of the foetus being able to mount a stress response and possibly being able to feel pain are profound and consideration must now be given to the provision of pain control for painful foetal interventions. General anaesthesia, opioids and local anaesthetics could be considered, either given directly to the foetus or by transplacental transfer. Long term consequences of foetal pain and stress on the structure and function of the developing nervous system are quite likely and may be prevented by analgesia.

PERINATAL STRESSES (BOXES 2.2–2.4)

The magnitude of the endocrine and metabolic changes noted above is several times less than those seen in babies during labour and vaginal delivery when very large rises in cortisol and catecholamines are seen. These are thought to be important in helping the

---

▼

Perinatal stresses

- pain
- cold
- undernutrition
- hypoglycaemia
- trauma
- hypovolaemia
- infection

Box 2.2

Neonatal risk factors for stress

- adaptation to extrauterine life
- limited endogenous reserves
- demands of growth
- immature organ function
- large body surface area
- congenital disorders
- low pain threshold
- infection

Box 2.3

**Painful and stressful procedures
in neonates**

- handling
- physiotherapy
- endotracheal suctioning
- tube feeding
- needling procedures
- capillary blood sampling
- chest drain insertion

Box 2.4

neonate adapt to extrauterine life, particularly in clearing the lungs of fluid, stimulating surfactant production, mobilizing glycogen and fat stores and maintaining blood flow to vital organs. So some stress is helpful. This can be illustrated, for example after a well-conducted Caesarean section delivery where the metabolic and hormonal changes in the baby are far less than after vaginal delivery. This situation is associated with more respiratory complications in the newborn period. In contrast, too much stress, or a normal amount of stress in a compromised baby, will be harmful.

The lower pain threshold to needling procedures is particularly relevant in clinical practice and the need to perform repeated heel-prick blood sampling results in marked sensitization of the baby's flexion-withdrawal reflex and obvious distress. The increase in variability of the heart rate, respiratory rate and oxygenation are quite good measures of the degree of this distress.

STRESS RESPONSE TO SURGERY

After surgery, the stress response is related to the severity of the surgical stimulus but also to the sickness of the baby beforehand. The sickest babies have higher catecholamine levels which result in a more marked hyperglycaemic response. Surgery results in release of peptides called cytokines and a whole series of catabolic hormones. Some of these hormonal changes may be designed to assist the healing process but extreme surgical stress is associated with increased morbidity and mortality. Ameliorating the stress by

---

▼ **Improving the perinatal stress response**

- suckling/feeding
- sucrose analgesia
- spring-loaded heel lance
- handling/massage
- environment: warmth; daylight–darkness cycle; noise reduction
- local and regional analgesia
- opioids
- general anaesthesia

Box 2.5

general, regional or opioid anaesthesia reduces morbidity and mortality (**Box 2.5**). The stress response does vary with gestational and postnatal age. The cortisol response is very short lived and attenuated in the pre-term baby and becomes more prolonged in older children. The noradrenaline response in neonates is significant and although an increase in adrenaline concentration occurs in neonates and young children, it is short lived, while in older children adrenaline rises are more persistent. Glucose metabolism and its control are disturbed by surgery but in an unpredictable way in neonates.

LONG TERM CONSEQUENCES OF NEONATAL PAIN OR EXPOSURE TO ANALGESICS

The neonatal peripheral and central nervous systems are quite different in structure, organization and function from the adult and this is reflected in the observed responses of the newborn baby to stimuli. The baby has a low threshold for responding and even non-noxious stimuli can produce a generalized exaggerated response which is poorly organized and localized. The response is often out of proportion to the stimulus and may last for a long time. Repeated stimuli may cause further lowering of the threshold for exaggerated responses and this is especially noticeable if the repeated stimuli are painful. The threshold is even lower if the tissues are damaged or inflamed and the nerve sprouting response may make the wound and surrounding area hypersensitive for many weeks. The gradual maturation and organization of excitatory and

27

inhibitory systems occurs over many weeks but may be profoundly affected by either untreated pain or by exposure to analgesics when not in pain. The long term consequences of untreated pain may be preventable by the provision of good analgesia. A good example is a study of neonatal circumcision (Taddio *et al.*, 1995) performed without analgesia where the pain threshold to subsequent vaccination was lowered for up to 6 months. If a local anaesthetic block was given to prevent the pain of circumcision, the subsequent lowering of the pain threshold did not occur. Twin studies have also shown behavioural differences later in life between the twin exposed to pain as a neonate compared with their sibling who had not experienced pain. On the other hand, it is now realized that use of analgesics in infants who are not in pain may also have long term effects which are undesirable. For example, those newborn animals exposed to morphine when not in pain need higher doses of morphine later in life to achieve pain control, which suggests that their opioid receptor systems have been profoundly altered. (This effect was not found when the animals had been given morphine to treat a painful wound.) We should be cautious therefore about using high doses of opioids for long periods (e.g. in critically ill infants in intensive care).

In older children there are also long term consequences of pain and stress in earlier life. The age at which these stresses occur, their severity and whether they have been repeated are important (Stevenson, 1995).

DEVELOPMENT OF THE BRAIN
AND EMOTIONAL RESPONSES

The cerebral cortex has one-thousand million neurones by 20 weeks gestation and thereafter the nerves grow and form increasing numbers of connections. Electrical activity can be detected from about 20 weeks and impulses are getting through to the cerebral cortex from around 28 weeks gestation. The connections to the higher centres mature during the remainder of the foetal period and this maturation continues for many years. The descending inhibitory pathways mature some time after birth, which may make the neonate hypersensitive to pain.

Emotional development affects the responses to painful stimuli in a profound way. In young children an all-or-nothing response to pain is seen and as their speech matures they increasingly complain when pain is present and ask why it is not being relieved. They can increasingly localize and describe pain intensity and its nature. Separation from parents greatly exaggerates responses to pain. After age five years, children increasingly can describe and grade their pain experience and describe it using analogies. They can be taught to use techniques to distract themselves from pain and can be taught to effectively control their own pain management. Their previous experiences of pain, the cultural, social and ethnic background and the context of the pain all have profound influences.

KEY LEARNING POINTS

- the developing nervous system is in a hyperexcitable state so that even non-noxious low threshold stimuli can produce a response

that is similar to that evoked by noxious stimuli, and repeated stimuli lower the threshold further
- opioid receptors are present and functional from early in development
- a metabolic and hormonal stress response is seen throughout development and occurs even in foetuses exposed to noxious stimuli
- early exposure to pain can profoundly affect subsequent behaviour and response to analgesics
- brain maturation and emotional development significantly affect pain behaviour and must be taken into account in methods of pain management

REFERENCES AND FURTHER READING

Aynsley-Green A. (1996) Pain and stress in infancy and childhood – where to now? *Paediatric Anaesthesia* **6**, 167–172.

Aynsley-Green A., Ward Platt M.P. and Lloyd-Thomas A.R. (1995) Stress and pain in infancy and childhood. *Bailliere's Clinical Paediatrics* **3**, 449–631.

Dickenson A.H. (1995) Spinal cord pharmacology of pain. *British Journal of Anaesthesia* **75**, 193–200.

Fitzgerald M. (1995) Developmental biology of inflammatory pain. *British Journal of Anaesthesia* **75**, 177–185.

Glover V. and Giannakoulpoulos (1995) Stress and pain in the fetus. *Bailliere's Clinical Paediatrics* **3**, 496.

Johnson R.W. (1997) Pain. *Care of the Critically Ill* **13**, 145–149.

Notcutt W.G. (1997) What makes acute pain chronic? *Current Anaesthesia and Critical Care* **8**, 55–61.

Stevenson J. (1995) Long-term sequelae of acute stress in early life. *Bailliere's Clinical Paediatrics* **3**, 619–631.

Taddio A., Goldbach M., Ipp M., Stevens B. and Koren G. (1995) Effect of neonatal circumcision on pain responses during vaccination in boys. *Lancet* **345**, 291–292.

Walco G.A., Cassidy R.C. and Schechter N.L. (1994) Pain, hurt and harm. The ethics of pain control in infants and children. *New England Journal of Medicine* **331**, 541–544.

Wolf A.R. (1993) Treat the babies, not their stress responses. *Lancet* **342**, 324–327.

CHAPTER 3

PAIN ASSESSMENT IN CHILDREN

Neil S. Morton

Pain assessment versus pain measurement

Pre-empting pain and pain prevention

Developmentally appropriate pain assessments

Pain scoring systems

Pain is difficult to measure in children and this has led to the production of many pain measurement tools and scores for neonates, infants and children. It is very difficult to see which measurement should be used for daily pain management of paediatric patients of various ages in the very different clinical settings of the general post-operative ward, day surgery unit, accident and emergency department, outpatient clinic or intensive care unit. The clinician needs a system which reliably tracks both the child's experience of pain and the efficacy of pain control over time. The researcher needs a tool that is rigorously proven for reliability in individual children when different observers are involved and for validity (i.e. the tool is actually measuring the child's pain and not something else). Many of the researcher's pain tools are too complicated, impractical and time consuming to be useful in clinical work.

PAIN ASSESSMENT VERSUS PAIN MEASUREMENT

Pain assessment is a broader concept than pain measurement. There are seven aspects of acute pain to be considered when assessing pain. Most pain measurement tools and scores try to assign a number to just one of these. Cognitive, physiological, sensory, behavioural, affective, sociocultural and environmental factors all affect pain assessment. The good doctor or nurse does include all these factors when caring for a child in pain and puts them together to individualize the child's management. Knowing the child's age, social circumstances and cultural background, a judgement of that particular child is made at that particular time in that particular medical environment having undergone a specific surgical procedure. Is the child exhibiting behavioural, physiological or emotional evidence of pain and if so how severe is it? What intervention is appropriate to try to control the pain? Having intervened, is the intervention adequate? If necessary further intervention is undertaken. This is the essence of the concept of *titration*. Staff may (almost unconsciously) compare this child with previous children they have cared for to judge whether they are following the anticipated path to recovery. Deviations from this anticipated path should be studied carefully and the reasons dealt with. Measurements with pain tools or scores should be regarded as an aid to this more complex overall assessment process (Beyer and Wells, 1989; Lloyd-Thomas, 1995).

Doctors and nurses who are caring for children need to be adequately trained to recognize acute pain in various age groups and must know how to intervene safely, effectively and appropriately to control pain. The classic scenario of the uncomplaining silent child who lies still and rigid after an abdominal operation scoring zero for pain at rest may seem like the ideal patient to inexperienced staff. The child may be terrified to move in case it hurts and may not complain in case he gets an intramuscular injection!

The aim is to get consistency of pain assessment built into daily clinical management while ensuring that assessments are not done for their own sake but are acted upon when required to optimize pain control for each individual child. Pain assessments must be regularly carried out and management adjusted regularly to maintain an acceptable level of pain control for that particular child. This individualized titration of analgesia can only be achieved by regular reassessment and re-evaluation of treatment (Beyer and Wells, 1989; Consumers' Association,1995; Lloyd-Thomas, 1995). After major paediatric surgery, *hourly* assessments of pain can easily be incorporated into the routine postoperative observations recorded by the nurse in the general ward, high dependency unit or intensive care unit (Morton, 1993). This is appropriate while the child is receiving complex analgesia with opioid infusions, PCA or epidural techniques (Lloyd-Thomas, 1995). Hourly re-evaluation of analgesic efficacy, adverse effects (sedation, respiratory depression, cardiovascular changes, emesis) and checks on the infusion device and delivery system should be routine. These observations may have to be increased in frequency if analgesia is poor or the patient is experiencing excessive adverse effects. Observations should be continued during and for some time after weaning from complex to simple analgesia. This has the advantages of firstly, making the nurse put the pain assessment into context for that child at that time and secondly, linking assessment to treatment. The pain assessment result should be recorded on an appropriate chart, preferably as part of the routine nursing charts or on a chart designed for that particular analgesic technique. The pain assessment becomes one component of a complete approach to the child which reduces the risk of staff focussing in on pain and its control to the exclusion of all else. For example, the restless child with cramping lower abdominal discomfort may have urinary retention and a full bladder, not wound pain.

After intermediate and minor surgery the frequency of observations can be reduced to 2 or 4 hourly, but pain assessment should be part of the routine nursing observations.

For paediatric day surgical cases, adequate pain control must be achieved before the child is discharged home and parents should be given clear instructions on how to assess and manage pain at home (McGrath *et al.*, 1994).

For every paediatric patient, a plan which incorporates prevention and control of pain, management of adverse effects, mobilization and restoration of function can be drawn up, thus integrating pain assessment and management into the overall care plan.

PRE-EMPTING PAIN AND PAIN PREVENTION

The pain assessment–intervention–reassessment cycle implies a reactive type of care but in very many paediatric situations the care has to be proactive, particularly as we know that many medical and nursing interventions are going to be painful. The problem is to get staff to think ahead and to prevent pain whenever possible.

Children hate injections, so avoiding intramuscular injections by using the intravenous, subcutaneous, rectal or oral routes of administration is extremely important. Using topical local anaesthetic creams (EMLA or amethocaine) routinely prior to all needling procedures in children is vital in breaking the culture of needle phobia and fear of injections in children. The use of local or regional anaesthesia as part of the technique for *all* painful procedures should be routine unless there is a specific reason not to. These techniques are proven to be highly effective.

Adequate loading and maintenance doses of opioids, NSAIDs and paracetamol should be prescribed and administered where appropriate. 'As-required' or 'prn' prescriptions should be avoided. In a busy hospital they are equivalent to writing 'I know this will not be given'! It is better to write timed doses to be given regularly so that therapeutic blood and tissue concentrations of the drug are maintained. These timed prescriptions are more likely to be given and are more effective in providing pain control. The timed prescription should be reviewed every 24 hours to ensure maximum dosage limits are not exceeded and to assess the need to continue each drug in the light of the assessment of pain control and adverse effects.

These techniques should be used together as multimodal analgesia, attacking the pain pathways at different points simultaneously. Adequate rescue analgesia and options for breakthrough pain must be available, with extra analgesia being given before physiotherapy, dressing changes or drain removals either by top-up bolus

37

doses or using techniques such as Entonox inhalation where appropriate. This *proactive* approach, reinforced by good patient and parental information delivered by well-educated staff, means putting pain control to the top of the list of priorities. Early pain-free mobilization and restoration of function is the aim.

To give this standard of care to all children whatever their age, medical and surgical status and wherever they are being looked after is difficult and requires coordination and cooperation amongst several disciplines. A pain management service or pain control team is the most efficient way to provide a comprehensive clinical service and can also undertake staff and patient education (Consumers' Association, 1995). The work of the pain control team should be audited regularly with research and development of new drugs and techniques forming the basis of improvements in the service.

DEVELOPMENTALLY APPROPRIATE PAIN ASSESSMENTS

Pain assessment is most accurate when the child can tell staff about their pain. They need to be given the opportunity, however, and this often does not happen in a busy hospital. For many reasons, children may not ask for pain relief, either because they do not want to disturb staff or because the remedy is unpleasant or induces adverse effects (e.g. IM injections of opioids).

It is possible for children down to the age of three years to *self-report* the location and severity of pain using words appropriate to their stage of development. Younger children cannot do so readily (Beyer and Wells, 1989). To pick up the symptoms and signs of pain in the younger child, more behavioural cues and physiological values are used. These are open to misinterpretation and can be affected by symptoms and events other than pain. It is important that staff are trained to detect the symptoms and signs of pain in different age groups and take a sufficiently broad view of the child to determine whether the observations they are making are caused by pain or by other factors. It is well established that experienced paediatric nurses are better at this than trainees and that parents can be better than nurses (Manne *et al.*, 1992).

NEONATES (UP TO I M; EX-PRETERM UP TO 60 WEEKS POST-CONCEPTUAL AGE)

In neonates, behaviours and physiological values are interpreted together to judge whether the baby is in distress and needs an analgesic intervention. What is often omitted, however, is reassessment of the effectiveness of the intervention in changing the pattern of behavioural and physiological changes. If this does not indicate improvement, then either the intervention may not have been adequate or the changes may not have been due to pain in the first place.

A variety of assessment tools have been developed and validated for neonates. Observation of facial expression, body position and movement, crying, blood pressure, heart rate, skin colour, oxygen saturation, respiratory rate and sleeplessness are all used. However, these can all be affected by non-painful things. A more useful assessment for clinical use is a more dynamic one, where improvement in the behavioural and physiological changes is sought in response to comforting, analgesia or sedation.

The younger, less mature, critically ill, sedated or

paralysed baby is unable to show the same pain behaviours as the healthy full term baby or older infant.
Many of the scoring systems do not work in the intubated ventilated neonate. Again by employing a dynamic
assessment of the response to nursing interventions such
as airway suctioning, a better estimate of depth of sedation and analgesia can be made. It is reasonable to
assume that the ventilated neonate will sense discomfort from the endotracheal tube, ventilatory support and
interventions such as suctioning, heel-prick blood sampling, insertion of intravascular lines and chest drain
insertion and removal. Adequate analgesia should be
given for these interventions in a pre-emptive way.
Continuous infusions of opioids can give rise to problems of tolerance, cumulation, withdrawal syndromes
and possibly immunosuppression. The longer term
effects of continuous exposure of the neonatal central
nervous system to opioids is not known and a better
option may be to consider short term infusions to cover
acutely painful episodes with regular reassessment
between infusions of the level of sedation and analgesia
required. Use of simple techniques such as 'sucrose
analgesia' (Ramenghi et al., 1996) and spring-loaded
capillary blood sampling systems are far safer and as
effective for painful procedures. With modern endotracheal tubes, fixation systems and synchronized or trig-
gered ventilatory modes, the discomfort from these
aspects of care is far less than with previous less sophis-
ticated systems. Neonates are sensitive to the sedative
and respiratory depressant effects of benzodiazepines
and opioids with longer elimination times leading to
cumulation on repeated dosing. Thus, non-ventilated
neonates require lower and less frequent doses and
very intensive monitoring when such agents are used.

INFANTS (1 M–1 Y) AND TODDLERS (1 Y–3 Y)

The same problems apply to infants. Metabolic systems are maturing rapidly in the first 3 months of life and renal function is maturing for the first year of life. The sedative and analgesic requirements may peak around the age of one year because of increased metabolic capacity and clearance. With adequate monitoring, conventional doses of analgesics and sedatives can be used safely in infants greater than 3 months of age and assessment of their effectiveness and adverse effects using behavioural and physiological responses is acceptable. The response to comforting measures and analgesic interventions should be documented. Remember, however, that exhibited behaviours may be less obvious in the very sick baby, or when ventilated, paralysed and sedated. In toddlers, exhibited behaviours may be more vigorous with an 'all-or-nothing' type of response. Sometimes the response is more precise, e.g. grabbing at the operation site if it is painful.

CHILDREN AGE 3–7 Y

Most 3 year olds can differentiate the presence or absence of pain. They can indicate pain intensity in up to four broad categories, corresponding to nil, mild, moderate and severe. Many can speak well enough to explain whether they are feeling pain and to indicate how bad it is (mild, moderate or severe), but using language and phrases they can understand. They can usually point to where the pain is. They can understand the concept of 'pieces of hurt' as used with the poker-chip tool (**Appendix 1**). The 'Faces' scale can work but younger children may think they have to choose the happiest face and do not relate the faces to their own pain experience (**Appendix 1**). Other younger children tend to choose at the extremes of such scales (i.e. an all-or-nothing effect). The faces scale works best if the choices are limited to four. Older children can also relate to previous pain experiences to indicate their current experience (e.g. from a cut or fall). The same tissue injury in a younger child with no previous pain experiences may be scored as severe while an older child who has had a worse pain before may score the pain as mild. Alternatively, children who have undergone repeated painful procedures may be sensitized and have very low pain thresholds. A more detailed faces progression using photographs arranged vertically (Oucher scale) can be used in this age group and ethically appropriate versions are available (Beyer and Wells, 1989). Visual analogue scales can be operated by children from around the age of 5 years but the classical 100 mm horizontal line (**Appendix 1**) is not well understood by younger children. Adding colour gradations is helpful and making the scale vertical, like a thermometer, is better understood (**Appendix 1**) (McGrath *et al.*, 1996).

OLDER CHILDREN AND ADOLESCENTS (7 Y+)

Older children can usually use visual or colour analogue scales and can self-report pain intensity, location and quality.

For severe or acute pain which is likely to last or need intervention over several days, the DEGR scale, which incorporates an assessment of the emotional or affective component (anxiety, depression) is useful (Gauvain-Piquard *et al.*, 1987).

PAIN SCORING SYSTEMS

In neonates, the CRIES score is easy to remember and works well in all but the very preterm and in the sedated

	Pain scoring systems

Neonate (0–1 m): behavioural and physiological signs of distress
OPS (Hannallah *et al.*, 1987; Broadman *et al.*, 1988; Norden *et al.*, 1991a,b)

advantages	● easy to use ● 5 categories ● validated against CHEOPS and Faces ● tracks pain over time and scores decrease with analgesia ● reliable between observers
disadvantages	● BP measurements may upset neonates ● cannot use in intubated paralysed babies ● 3 out of 5 categories are similar

CRIES (Krechel and Bildner, 1995)

advantages	● easy to remember and use ● valid and reliable down to 32 w gestational age ● reliable between observers ● tracks pain and the effect of analgesics
disadvantages	● uses oxygenation as a measure which can be affected by many other factors ● BP measurement may upset baby

NIPS (Lawrence *et al.*, 1993)

disadvantages	● uses 6 categories, 2 of which are similar ● hard to remember ● cannot be used in intubated or paralysed patients

COMFORT (Ambuel *et al.*, 1992)

disadvantages	● complicated ● 8 categories and many subcategories ● cannot be used in intubated or paralysed patients

CHEOPS (McGrath *et al.,* 1985)

    disadvantages
- complicated behavioural scale
- may not track post-operative pain well in 3–7 year olds as pain behaviour inhibited

Barrier et al., 1989

    disadvantages
- 10 categories, 4 of which are similar
- confusing (high score = low pain)
- cannot be used in intubated or paralysed patients

Infant and toddler (1 m–3 y): behavioural and physiological signs of distress
OPS
COMFORT
CHEOPS
TPPPS (Tarbell *et al.,* 1992)

    advantages
- suitable for age 1–5 y
- tracks pain relief and effects of analgesics
- correlates with nurse and parental pain assessments

    disadvantages
- 7 categories to score

Nurse observations (Manne *et al.,* 1992)

    advantages
- easy to incorporate into routine observations
- experienced nurse usually accurate

    disadvantages
- observer bias
- lack of training leads to inaccuracy

Parental observations (Manne *et al.,* 1992; McGrath *et al.,* 1994)
- parental observations often accurate and helpful

Children (3 y–7 y): behavioural and physiological signs of distress plus self-reporting
OPS
COMFORT

CHEOPS
TPPPS
FACES SCALE (Beyer and Wells, 1989)

- younger children tend to choose extremes
- best with 4 choices
- some children confuse with happiness measure

POKER CHIP TOOL (Beyer and Wells, 1989)
COLOUR SCALES (Beyer and Wells, 1989)
OUCHER (Beyer and Wells, 1989)
HORIZONTAL LINEAR ANALOGUE (Beyer and Wells, 1989)
VERTICAL LINEAR ANALOGUE (Beyer and Wells, 1989)
COLOURED VERTICAL ANALOGUE (McGrath et al., 1996)

- age 5 y+
- very easy to use

DEGR (Gauvain-Piquard et al., 1987)

- for longer lasting pain
- takes into account anxiety and depression

ADJECTIVAL SELF-REPORT (Morton, 1993)

- easy to use
- 4 categories sensitive enough to track pain and effect of analgesics
- use language that the child can understand

Children (7y +): self-report
COLOURED VERTICAL ANALOGUE
HORIZONTAL LINEAR ANALOGUE
ADJECTIVAL SELF-REPORT

Box 3.1

paralysed ventilated baby. In infants and toddlers, the OPS is easy to use and the TPPPS, although more complex, has been found to track pain intensity and control pain well. From age 3 years, children can self report the presence of pain and grade its intensity, although younger children tend to do this as an all-or-nothing response. Self-reporting with words or visual aids is sensitive enough to track pain control, provided the number of choices is limited to around 4 words, faces or 'pieces of hurt'. Linear analogues are understood from around age 5 years and colour-graded vertical scales seem to be the most practical. However, verbal self-reporting also works well. From age 7 years, the classical horizontal VAS can work but the vertical colour analogue scale and self reporting are also reliable. Whichever scoring system is used, the assessments should be repeated regularly, appropriate interventions should be prescribed and their effectiveness in reducing the pain score should be regularly documented.

KEY LEARNING POINTS

- all children should be regularly assessed for the presence of pain, its intensity and its cause using a method of assessment appropriate to the child's stage of development and severity of illness
- titration of pain control against regular reassessments is the best way to control pain
- documentation of the efficacy and adverse effects of pain management should be routine in all age groups and in all medical environments
- pain assessment tools can help to track the need for analgesia and whether it has been effective
- pain control should be continuous throughout the hospital stay, including the period of mobilization and return to function, and arrangements should be made for continuing pain control at home if appropriate

REFERENCES AND FURTHER READING

Ambuel B., Hamlett K.W., Marx C.M. and Plummer J.L. (1992) Assessing distress in pediatric intensive care environments. The COMFORT scale. *Journal of Pediatric Psychology* **17**, 95–109.

Barrier G., Attia J., Mayer M.N., Amiel-Tison C.L. and Schnider S.M. (1989) Measurement of postoperative pain and narcotic administration in infants using a new clinical scoring system. *Intensive Care Medicine* **15**, S37–S39.

Beyer J.E. and Wells N. (1989) The assessment of pain in children. *Pediatric Clinics of North America* **36**, 837–853.

Beyer J.E., McGrath P.J. and Berde C.B. (1990) Discordance between self-report and behavioural pain measures in children aged 3–7 years after surgery. *Journal of Pain and Symptom Management* **5**, 350–356.

Broadman L.M., Rice L.H. and Hannallah R.S. (1988) Testing the validity of an objective pain scale for infants and children. *Anesthesiology* **69**, A770.

Consumers' Association (1995) Managing acute pain in children. *Drugs and Therapeutics Bulletin* **33**, 41–44.

Gauvain-Piquard A., Rodary C., Rezvani A. and Lemerle J. (1987) Pain in children aged 2–6 years: a new observational rating scale elaborated in a pediatric oncology unit – preliminary report. *Pain* **31**, 177–188.

Hannallah R.S., Broadman L.M., Belman A.S., Abramowitz M.D. and Epstein B.S. (1987) Comparison of caudal and ilioinguinal/ iliohypogastric nerve blocks for control of post orchiopexy pain in pediatric ambulatory surgery. *Anesthesiology* **66**, 832–834.

Krechel S.W. and Bildner J. (1995) CRIES: a new neonatal postoperative pain measurement score. Initial testing of validity and reliability. *Paediatric Anaesthesia* **5**, 53–61.

Lawrence J., Alcock D., McGrath P., Kay J., MacMurray S.B. and Dulberg C. (1993) The development of a tool to assess neonatal pain. *Neonatal Network* **12**, 59–65.

Lloyd-Thomas A. (1995) Assessment and control of pain in children. *Anaesthesia* **50**, 753–755.

Manne S.L., Jacobsen P.B. and Redd W.H. (1992) Assessment of acute pediatric pain: do child self report, parent rating and nurse ratings measure the same phenomena? *Pain* **48**, 45–52.

McGrath P.A., Seifert C.E., Speechley K.N., Booth J.C., Stitt L. and Gibson M.C. (1996) A new analogue scale for assessing children's pain: an initial validation study. *Pain* **64**, 435–443.

McGrath P.J., Johnson G., Goodman J.T., Schillinger J., Dunn J. and Chapman J.A. (1985) CHEOPS: a behavioural scale for rating postoperative pain in children. *Advances in Pain Research and Therapy* **9**, 395–402.

McGrath P.J., Finley G.A. and Ritchie J. (1994) Parents' roles in pain assessment and management. *IASP Newsletter* **March/April**, 3–4.

McGrath P.J., Unruh A.M. and Finley G.A. (1995) Pain measurement in children. *IASP Pain Clinical Updates* **3**, 1–4.

Morton N.S. (1993) Development of a monitoring protocol for the safe use of opioids in children. *Paediatric Anaesthesia* **3**, 179–184.

Norden J., Hannallah R., Getson P., O'Donnell R., Kelliher G. and Walker N. (1991a) Concurrent validation of an objective pain scale for infants and children. *Anesthesiology* **75**, A934.

Norden J., Hannallah R., Getson P., O'Donnell R., Kelliher G. & Walker N. (1991b) Reliability of an objective pain scale in children. *Anesthesia and Analgesia* **72**, S199.

Ramenghi L.A., Wood C.M., Griffith G.C. & Levene M.I. (1996) Reduction of pain response in premature infants using intraoral sucrose. *Archives of Disease in Childhood Fetal and Neonatal Edition* **74**, F126–F128.

Tarbell S.E., Cohen I.T. and Marsh J.L. (1992) The Toddler-Preschooler Postoperative Pain Scale: an observational scale for measuring postoperative pain in children aged 1–5. Preliminary report. *Pain* **50**, 273–280.

CHAPTER 4

PHARMACOLOGY OF ANALGESICS IN CHILDREN

Tom G. Hansen, Steen W. Henneberg

Practical paediatric pharmacology

Local anaesthetics

Opioid analgesics

Non-opioid analgesics

During the last decade our understanding of the pharmacology of analgesics in children older than 1 year of age has increased, but is less comprehensive in the youngest age groups. Children differ from adults in the way they respond to drugs and this especially applies to neonates and premature infants. Several changes occur during development which affect the dose, route and duration of analgesic use. New information about an analgesic is almost always collected after the drug has undergone adult trials and is often incomplete even after the drug has started to be used in paediatrics. Ethical principles suggest that new drugs should be used and evaluated first in adults but this approach may delay proper paediatric studies, especially neonatal ones. The lack of methods for drug analysis in small plasma or blood samples can be a problem and there are ethical limitations on how much blood can be taken from the child for such studies, for example limits suggested are 1ml/kg (maximum 10 ml) or 1–5% of the blood volume.

PRACTICAL PAEDIATRIC PHARMACOLOGY

The study of the processing of drugs by the body is called *pharmacokinetics* while the study of the effects of drugs on the body is called *pharmacodynamics*.

PROCESSING OF DRUGS BY THE BODY

Absorption

In children the most common routes of administration of analgesics are oral, rectal or intravenous (iv). The subcutaneous (sc, under the skin), epidural (into the epidural space), intrathecal (into the cerebrospinal fluid in the subarachnoid space), transdermal (via the skin) and transmucosal (nasal, sublingual, lingual or buccal) routes are used less commonly and intramuscular (im) injections are to be avoided unless absolutely necessary. This is because *children hate injections*!

Most orally ingested drugs are absorbed from the upper part of the small intestine and some from the gastric mucosa. The hydrogen ion concentration of the stomach and intestine, the rate of gastric emptying and the physical and chemical properties of the drug determine the amount of absorption. The stomach is relatively alkaline in the neonate (i.e. the hydrogen ion concentration is relatively low) but there is considerable variation. Adult levels are reached at the age of 3 years. Gastric emptying time is prolonged in younger infants and in fact is inversely related to gestational maturity and post-natal age. Thus, the less mature and younger the baby, the more prolonged is gastric emptying. Drugs absorbed from the gastrointestinal mucosa pass via the portal venous system to the liver and often undergo a considerable degree of metabolism during their first circulation through the liver tissue. This 'first-pass' metabolism will result in much less drug reaching the systemic circulation. The combination of gastric alkalinity, slow gastric emptying and high first-pass liver extraction of orally administered drugs means that a relatively high dose has to be given by this route to achieve therapeutic plasma, central nervous system and tissue concentrations equivalent to those achieved by intravenous administration.

Rectal administration of drugs has been popular in paediatrics, and this route may be useful under circumstances where the oral route cannot be used, for example following major surgery or when the child is fasted or nauseated. There is less surface area available for absorption of drugs from the rectum than from the upper gastrointestinal tract. Rectal absorption is variable and unpredictable. Some children find this route unpleasant and consent should be sought from the child and the parents. Rectal absorption is influenced by a number of different factors such as: faecal content, hydrogen ion concentration, formulation of the drug and site of placement of the drug in the rectum. If the drug is placed too high in the rectum, it will be absorbed directly into the portal circulation and will go straight to the liver. A large proportion of the dose will be metabolized resulting in a low systemic plasma and tissue concentration. If the drug is given low in the rectum, it will be absorbed into venous blood draining via the middle and inferior rectal veins and thus bypass the first-pass metabolism in the liver. This can be a very efficient way of giving drugs such as diclofenac which reaches a peak plasma concentration within 30 minutes of rectal administration.

Subcutaneous administration of analgesics, as bolus

doses and/or continuous infusions, can be very useful in children, particularly after orthopaedic surgery. This obviates the need for maintaining venous access for several days. A small cannula is sited either during general anaesthesia or under topical local anaesthesia of the skin. The cannula is best placed centrally, for example over the anterior abdominal wall, upper anterior chest wall, deltoid region of the upper arm or lateral aspect of the thigh. Delayed and variable absorption may be expected by this route if the peripheral circulation is poor, for example in the child who is cold or has reduced circulating volume. This route should not be used in such cases as the subcutaneous depot of drug will be washed out into the child's circulation when the peripheral skin blood flow is restored to normal upon rewarming or fluid resuscitation. Usually a smaller volume of more concentrated drug solution is given subcutaneously than when the same dose is given intravenously so that there is less injection pain.

Although the absorption of a drug is faster and less variable following intramuscular injection, this route of administration should rarely be needed in paediatrics. An intramuscular cannula can, however, be sited while the child is undergoing general anaesthesia which can be used in the same way as a subcutaneous cannula and may be associated with less stinging on injection of bolus doses. The limitations noted above for the subcutaneous route also apply to the intramuscular route.

After intravenous administration, the drug is available immediately and the first pass extraction by the liver does not apply. The intravenous dose required to achieve a given effect is therefore much lower than the oral dose. Normally intravenous doses are given as dilute solutions, slowly in fractionated increments with intervals between each small incremental dose to see the effect. This is called *titration*.

Ionization

Most analgesics are present in plasma in both ionized (charged) and non-ionized (uncharged) forms. The non-ionized form of the drug crosses the phospholipid layer of biological membranes more readily. The acidity or alkalinity of the local environment determines how a given drug behaves. For example, in acidic environments such as the stomach, most of a weak acid is present in the non-ionized, readily absorbable form, whereas weak bases will be in the ionized, poorly absorbable form.

Distribution

Having reached the circulation, the distribution of a drug around the body is influenced by a number of age-dependent factors. The composition of the body in terms of fluid and fat, the location of fluid compartments in the body and their size, the cardiac output and the local blood flow are all important. Drug-specific factors such as fat solubility and protein binding also affect distribution.

Protein binding

A substantial number of analgesics are bound to plasma proteins (albumin, alpha-1-acid glycoprotein and gamma-globulins). Only the free, unbound portion of the drug is pharmacologically active and available to reach target organs and for metabolism. In a sense, the protein-bound portion is a depot of the drug. Most opioids and local anaesthetics are bound by alpha-1–acid glycoprotein. The protein binding capacity in neonates and infants is low owing to both a reduced concentration of plasma proteins, and a reduced affinity for drugs. Furthermore, increased concentrations of free fatty acids and unconjugated bilirubin compete with acidic drugs for protein binding sites. Acidosis or alkalosis can also cause an increase in free unbound drugs.

Body fluid compartments

Body composition varies with age. Neonates and premature infants have more total body water and less muscle mass compared to children and adults. Total fat content of premature infants is even lower than in neonates (**Table 4.1**).

This means that water-soluble drugs are more widely distributed in the more extensive fluid compartments of small infants and thus a higher initial dose is required to achieve sufficient plasma and tissue concentrations. Theoretically the elimination should be prolonged owing to the larger volume of distribution, but this is often compensated by faster clearance, particularly in infants and toddlers. The distribution volume is mainly due to the properties of the drug, protein binding and tissue binding. A large distribution volume reflects

Table 4.1 **Body composition at different ages as percentage of body weight**

Age group	Total body water (%)	Extracellular water (%)	Fat (%)
Premature	85	50	<10
Neonate	78	45	12
Infant (1 y)	60	27	30
Adolescent	50	20	10–30[a]

[a] the fat content is higher on average in females at 20–30% compared with 10–15% in males

extensive uptake and tissue binding, for example fat-soluble drugs and those with low protein binding have a large volume of distribution. Renal, hepatic or cardiac failure, hypovolaemia or dehydration alter the distribution volume of drugs. In neonates during and after major surgery, hypovolaemia and dehydration may significantly alter drug kinetics. On a weight basis the cardiac output in a neonate is twice that of an older child (200 ml/kg/min versus 100 ml/kg/min), which means that most drugs are distributed to and from their sites of action more rapidly. The brain in newborns and infants is relatively large and it receives a greater percentage of the cardiac output than in adults. The neonatal brain is thus a significant target organ for lipid-soluble drugs. In the premature neonate the ability to redistribute these drugs to muscle or fat tissue is limited.

Elimination

Elimination includes all the processes responsible for the removal of a drug from the body. Liver metabolism and excretion via the kidneys are the most important. A measurement of elimination of a drug is the *clearance*, which is the volume of blood per minute from which drug is removed and is usually corrected for body weight or body surface area.

Metabolism

The main sites of metabolism of drugs are the liver microsomal enzyme system, plasma esterases, kidneys and the lungs. Liver metabolism either causes *degradation* of drugs by oxidation, reduction or hydrolysis or *synthesis* of water-soluble compounds which are more easily excreted via the kidneys. These synthetic reactions are forms of conjugation (glucuronidation, sulphation, methylation and acetylation). The newer opioids such as fentanyl, alfentanil and sufentanil are degraded. In most cases the biotransformation leads to inactivation of the drug. Sometimes, however, the metabolites are active, e.g. morphine is metabolized to both morphine-3-glucuronide (which has anti-analgesic and stimulatory properties) and morphine-6-glucuronide (which is a potent, long-acting analgesic). In neonates, the concentration and activity of enzyme systems is less than in adults, because of the immaturity of the liver at this stage of development. The synthetic reactions are more affeceted by this immaturity. Glucuronide conjugation, for example, does not reach adult values until the age of 3 months. In the neonatal period, hepatic clearance is the most important factor influencing the biodisposition of analgesics. Hepatic blood flow and metabolism undergo substantial changes in neonates. The ductus venosus, which bypasses the hepatic circulation, leads to decreased hepatic blood flow and hence drug metabolism. The ductus venosus closes at 2–3 weeks of postnatal age and by that time the portal vein becomes a significant contributor to hepatic blood flow, making entero-hepatic recirculation possible. The kidneys are also immature in the neonate and have less ability to concentrate substances for excretion in the urine. The overall effect of these differences is that in the neonate, the elimination of drugs is significantly delayed.

However, the clearance of most drugs improves within the first month of life. In the infant, the capacity to metabolize drugs, particularly by degradation reactions, is markedly increased. From age 1–5 years, children eliminate lipid-soluble drugs 2–6 times quicker than older children and adults! From 3 months of age onwards the relative metabolic rate of degradative reactions increases to a maximum by age 2–3 years. The liver is relatively large in these young children (4% of body weight compared with 2% in the adult) and there is a relatively large liver blood flow. The overall effect is to shorten the effect of bolus doses of analgesics.

The biotransformation of some drugs involves esterases present in plasma, on red blood cells and in different tissues. Reduced activity of pseudocholinesterase, acetylcholinesterase and arylesterase have been found in preterm neonates which may result in a prolonged effect of ester analgesics. The esterase activity gradually increases during the first year of life, paralleling the increase seen in plasma protein concentrations. Amethocaine and remifentanil are examples of analgesics which are cleared by esterase degradation and care may be needed with use of these drugs in preterm neonates.

Excretion

The main route of drug excretion is via the kidneys. The number of nephrons is the same in neonates as in adults but they are neither anatomically nor functionally mature until the age of 6 months. In the neonatal period, the glomerular filtration rate (GFR) is low (0.7–4.0 ml/min) but increases subsequently during the following 10–20 weeks to adult values owing to increased renal blood flow and mean blood pressure as well as surface area and permeability of the membrane of Bowman's capsule. Similarly, tubular function matures to adult levels within the first year. Hence, glomerular function matures more rapidly than tubular function. At a certain point this imbalance may result in a higher clearance of various compounds than seen in older children. Overall, delayed elimination of most analgesic metabolites is seen in the first 6 months of life. The relative capacity of the kidneys to excrete drugs increases steadily to a maximum by age 2–3 years.

Pulmonary excretion

Nitrous oxide and volatile anaesthetics are primarily excreted through the lungs. The rate of excretion depends mainly on the inspired fraction of the gas and the alveolar ventilation.

EFFECTS OF ANALGESICS ON THE BODY

Analgesics act via cell membrane receptors, ion channels and intra-membrane pumps primarily in the central nervous system. The delivery of a drug to its receptor is dependent on dose and time. Age, maturity and diseases can affect the numbers, types, availability and affinity of receptors. This seems particularly important in the neonatal period (see Chapter 2).

In normal children and adults the brain capillaries are relative impermeable to most ionized and water-soluble molecules. In the neonate the blood–brain barrier is poorly developed allowing ionized and water-soluble drugs to penetrate as easily as lipid-soluble compounds. The nerve fibres in neonates have less myelin coating so may be more susceptible to the effects of drugs such as local anaesthetics.

LOCAL ANAESTHETICS

Local anaesthetics should be part of the pain relief technique for all children unless there is a specific reason for not using them. This is because they have been proven to be so effective when used correctly.

MECHANISM OF ACTION

Local anaesthetics bind to receptor sites in the sodium channels of nerve fibres. This stops the influx of sodium and thus blocks conduction of impulses along the nerve. They are applied as near to the nerve tissue to be blocked as possible because they must cross the nerve cell membrane to access the sodium channels from the inside of the nerve.

CHEMISTRY

Local anaesthetics are composed of a lipid-soluble and a water-soluble part, separated by a hydrocarbon chain attached by either an ester group (-COO-) or an amide group (-CONH-). All local anaesthetics can be divided into two major groups according to the nature of this bond, namely esters and amides. For clinical use local anaesthetics are dispensed as a water-soluble hydro-chloride salt. In this solution there is an equilibrium of unionized and ionized local anaesthetic molecules. The unionized local anaesthetic is lipid soluble and can thus cross the nerve cell membrane easily. The potency of a local anaesthetic is related to its lipid solubility. How-ever, the ionized acid is the active substance in terms of blocking nerve conduction. The duration of action depends on the extent of protein binding, tissue uptake and affinity for neural tissue. The speed of onset depends on the dose and concentration of local anaes-thetic solution and the proportion that is in the active, ionized form at the target site. The equilibrium of local anaesthetic solution can be shifted towards more ionized acid by acidosis, for example in infected tissue. This will mean that there is plenty of the pharmacologically active form of the drug but it cannot reach the sodium channels because it cannot diffuse through the nerve cell membrane.

ABSORPTION

Following an injection of local anaesthetic, some diffuses into the nerve fibres but some is also taken up into the surrounding blood vessels. The amount of absorption into the circulation depends on the local numbers and size of the capillary vessels, cardiac output and regional blood flow, the affinity of the drug for blood compared with tissue (the blood/tissue partition coefficient) and the use of vasoconstrictors added to the local anaesthetic solution (e.g. adrenaline, noradrenaline, octapressin). Some local anaesthetics have inherent vasoconstrictor properties, e.g. cocaine. The absorption of a local anaesthetic is very fast following intercostal, interpleural or topical application to mucosal surfaces because these are very vascular sites. Whatever the intended site of administration, even a small dose given directly into a vein or an artery may produce toxic effects because a transient high peak concentration of local anaesthetic will reach the brain or heart muscle with possible toxic effects. Under normal circumstances 60–80% of an injected local anaesthetic dose is absorbed during the first passage in the lungs which protects against toxic reactions. This is well illustrated in some children with congenital heart defects involving shunting of blood from the lung circulation to the systemic circulation in whom the lungs are bypassed and a rapid, very high peak plasma concentration will occur. The lungs are easily saturated and this is important when a continuous infusion is being used.

PROTEIN BINDING

Local anaesthetics are bound primarily to alpha-1-acid glycoprotein (AAG), but also to albumin and gamma-globulins. For example, 65–70% of lignocaine and 95% of bupivacaine are bound to plasma proteins. The unbound part is the active drug in terms of both desirable and undesirable effects. The amount of plasma proteins and their binding capacity are reduced in neonates and there is a risk of high unbound local anaesthetic concentrations occurring in this age group particularly once all the binding sites are occupied, for example after several hours of continuous infusion at high rates. Bupivacaine has a low hepatic extraction ratio (low percentage of drug removed during one passage through the liver) and a high volume of distribution, particularly in neonates. This leads to a much prolonged half-life of bupivacaine in neonates. Liver enzyme immaturity is particularly important but reduction in liver blood flow or liver failure would cause free levels of bupivacaine to rise much more quickly leading to toxicity. Although the protein binding capacity of the neonate is reduced, the amount of free, unbound drug circulating is very small indeed and is usually within the clearance capability of the liver after single doses. Repeated doses, large doses, intravascular injection or continuous infusion could lead to free concentrations which exceed the liver's capacity to cope. Levels of binding proteins, especially alpha-1-acid glycoprotein, usually rise after surgery as part of the stress response to surgery. In very ill or preterm babies, however, this rise may not occur and these babies may have very low levels of binding proteins before surgery. Also, in sick neonates bilirubin may compete with bupivacaine for protein binding sites, displacing it and increasing the free concentration transiently.

METABOLISM

The metabolism of amide local anaesthetics is reduced in the neonate because liver enzyme systems are immature and liver blood flow is reduced. Enzyme immaturity is more important for those local anaesthetics with low hepatic extraction ratios such as bupivacaine. Reduction in liver blood flow is more important for those local anaesthetics with intermediate to high hepatic extraction ratios, such as lignocaine. The amides undergo dealkylation, hydroxylation and conjugation in the liver. In neonates the conjugation step (glucuronidation catalysed by the enzyme uridine diphosphate (UDP) glycuronyl transferase) has a considerably reduced activity. Overall, bupivacaine's metabolism is impaired more than that of lignocaine in the neonate because enzyme immaturity is more marked than the reduction in liver blood flow (**Table 4.2**).

The clearance of bupivacaine is reduced in neonates compared to older children and adults. With a larger volume of distribution, this results in a considerably prolonged elimination. The clearance of lignocaine seems to be age independent while the distribution

Table 4.2 **Pharmacokinetic variables for bupivacaine and lignocaine in neonates and older children**

Drug	Age group	Clearance (ml/kg/min)	Distribution volume (l/kg)	Elimination half-life (h)
Bupivacaine	Neonate	7	3.9	6–22
	Child	10	2.7	2–4
Lignocaine	Neonate	10	3.0	3.0
	Child	10	2.5	1.4

volume is greater in neonates resulting in a longer elimination time.

Prilocaine is metabolized in the liver to ortho-toluidine. This substance may inhibit the methaemoglobin reductase complex. In neonates, the activity of this complex is reduced and furthermore, foetal haemoglobin (HbF) is more easily transformed into methaemoglobin than adult haemoglobin (HbA). All together this renders the neonate more susceptible to prilocaine-induced methaemoglobinaemia and so care must be taken with prilocaine containing products such as EMLA cream in neonates, particularly as this product is more easily absorbed through immature skin.

The ester local anaesthetics such as amethocaine are hydrolysed by esterase enzymes in plasma, on red blood cells and in the tissues. Neonatal levels of these enzymes are somewhat reduced but there is usually sufficient capacity to cope with conventional doses of ester local anaesthetics.

OPIOID ANALGESICS

The naturally occurring alkaloids derived from opium are the opiates while synthetic compounds with morphine-like effects are opioids.

MECHANISM OF ACTION

The opioids exert their effect by binding to opioid receptors primarily located in the brain and spinal cord. However, opioid receptors have also been demonstrated outside the CNS, e.g. the lungs, adrenal glands, placenta, urinary and gastrointestinal tracts and on the surface of leucocytes, as well as on the peripheral end of primary afferent neurons. So far, five different opioid receptors have been demonstrated: mu1, mu2, kappa, delta and sigma (**Box 4.1**). In terms of analgesia, the mu-receptors are the most important receptors; the mu_1-receptor mediates supraspinal analgesia, whereas the mu_2-receptor mediates spinal analgesia and respiratory depression. The sigma-receptor is currently not recognized as a 'true' opioid receptor, because sigma-receptor mediated effects are not reversed by opioid antagonists. The body produces its own natural opioids: the enkephalins, endorphins and dynorphins, which act at these receptors in response to pain and stress.

ABSORPTION

Opioids are usually given by intravenous, intramuscular or subcutaneous injection but can be given orally or rectally. Lipid-soluble opioids such as fentanyl can also be absorbed through the skin (transdermal delivery) or from the oral mucosa (lingual, sublingual, oral transmucosal delivery). First-pass clearance by the liver is

Opioid receptors and their effects	
Receptor	Effect
mu_1	supraspinal analgesia, physical dependence, euphoria
mu_2	spinal analgesia, inhibition of gastrointestinal motility, respiratory depression, bradycardia, sedation, pupillary constriction, nausea and vomiting
kappa	spinal analgesia, sedation, pupillary constriction, inhibition of ADH production, dysphoria
delta	spinal analgesia, euphoria, respiratory depression
sigma	psychotomimetic effects (dysphoria and hallucinations), pupillary dilatation

Box 4.1

significant for oral administration, e.g. for morphine up to 80% of an oral dose undergoes first pass metabolic clearance and so oral doses have to be increased. This is discussed in more detail in Chapter 6.

METABOLISM

Glucuronidation in the liver is the main metabolic route for opioids and the glucuronidation capacity varies with gestational age. Sulphation plays a more minor role. Hepatic clearance is mature by about age 3 months. Renal excretion of these water soluble metabolites may initially be very low in the newborn but rapidly matures in the first few months and by age 1 year both glomerular and tubular function are mature. Doses of opioids usually need to be reduced in neonates by about 75%, but by age 3 months conventional doses corrected for body weight may be employed provided adequate monitoring is used (see Chapter 6).

In general the volume of distribution of morphine is unchanged at all ages whereas the half-life decreases as the clearance increases with age.

Using morphine as an illustration (**Table 4.3**), on average the volume of distribution is independent of age. The elimination half-life is markedly prolonged in preterm neonates and in all age groups a wide interindividual variation in clearance is seen (up to 7–fold).

Table 4.3 Pharmacokinetics of morphine at different ages

Age	Volume of distribution (l/kg)	Clearance (ml/min/kg)	Elimination half-life (h)
Preterm	2.8	2.2	9
Term neonate	2.8	8	6.5
Infant	2.8	24	2

NON-OPIOID ANALGESICS

PARACETAMOL

Paracetamol remains the most popular and widely used paediatric analgesic and antipyretic. Paracetamol can be given orally, rectally and intravenously (as the prodrug propacetamol, at present not available in the UK). The drug has a high therapeutic index, with an antipyretic plasma concentration range of 10–20 mg/l, as compared to plasma levels 6–10 times higher than these four hours after ingestion to produce toxicity (120 mg/l). The 'analgesic' plasma concentration range has never been established and there is little data concerning the analgesic efficacy of paracetamol in children. The analgesic potency probably corres-ponds to that of the NSAIDs. Paracetamol, like other NSAIDs, has a ceiling effect, so that for a further increase in dose no additional analgesia is seen.

Mechanism of action

Paracetamol is thought to work as an inhibitor of central nervous system prostaglandin synthesis but is only weakly anti-inflammatory.

Absorption and distribution

Absorption of paracetamol from the upper small intestine is rapid and almost complete (90%), whereas following rectal administration the bioavailability is only 40–80% of that of an oral dose. To achieve and maintain therapeutic plasma levels, a higher dose must be given rectally than orally (40 mg/kg versus 20 mg/kg) and the dosage interval for rectal administration should be longer than for the oral route (6 hours versus 4 hours). In neonates and infants the time to reach maximum plasma levels (T_{max}) following oral and rectal administration is about 60–90 minutes, while in older children it is 120 minutes after oral intake and 150 minutes after rectal administration. The volume of distribution and total body clearance of paracetamol are unknown in neonates and infants. In children > 3 years, the distribution volume is 0.80–0.95 l/kg and the clearance is 0.30–0.40 l/kg/hr. The elimination half-life in older children is 2–3 hours, slightly shorter in infants (1½–2 hours) and prolonged in neonates (3½–5 hours). The extent of plasma protein binding of paracetamol is unknown in neonates. In older children and adults levels of 15–25% have been reported.

Metabolism

Normally paracetamol is excreted by the kidneys after hepatic glucuronidation and sulphation. Less than 5% of the unchanged drug is recovered in the urine. Neonates, infants and children up to 9 years of age seem to metabolize paracetamol through sulphation rather than glucuronidation.

Side effects

Paracetamol has hardly any side effects when used in therapeutic concentrations, with occasional nausea and vomiting the only ones of note. A small proportion of paracetamol is metabolized by the cytochrome P450 system to form the potentially hepatotoxic metabolite N-acetyl-p-benzoquinoneimine (NABQI). This metabolite is normally inactivated by conjugation with hepatic glutathione to produce a non-toxic metabolite which is excreted in the urine. If a large amount of this metabolite is produced following large doses of paracetamol, hepatic glutathione deposits may be depleted and reaction of NABQI with hepatic proteins increases. This may lead to hepatic necrosis. Neonates and infants have higher hepatic glutathione levels and lower cytochrome P450 activities, and hence they are partially protected from these toxic effects of paracetamol.

NON-STEROIDAL ANTI-INFLAMMATORY DRUGS (NSAIDS)

The non-steroidal anti-inflammatory drugs have been used with increasing frequency in paediatrics in the treatment of pain. The NSAIDs have mainly been used in juvenile rheumatoid arthritis but during the last decade also in post-operative pain management in children. For mild to moderate pain the NSAIDs may be used as a sole agent or combined with local anaesthetics or opioids. Following minor surgery (e.g. dental, ENT or minor general surgery) efficacy has been demonstrated by a reduction in pain score when used alone or in conjunction with different regional anaesthetic techniques. When used instead of opioids fewer side effects may be encountered. Following major surgery, the use of NSAIDs lowers the dose of opioids needed to achieve satisfactory pain control, i.e. an 'opioid-sparing' effect. Theoretically, this should also reduce the freqency of opioid-related side effects.

The NSAIDs act through an inhibition of prostaglandin synthesis in the tissues. Arachidonic acid derived from cell membranes in connection with trauma or inflammation is metabolized either to prostaglandins and thromboxane A_2 via the cyclo-oxygenase pathway or to leukotrienes via the lipo-oxygenase pathway. The prostaglandins and thromboxane A_2 are potent vasodilators and inflammatory mediators, synergizing with other molecules such as bradykinin and histamine.

Leukotrienes are potent bronchoconstrictors. The NSAIDs mainly inhibit the cyclo-oxygenase pathway reducing the tissue inflammatory response and reducing the production of pain producing substances from injured tissues. This results in a switching of arachidonic acid metabolism towards leukotriene production and this may explain the aggravation of bronchospasm in some asthmatics who receive NSAIDs.

Absorption and distribution

Following oral administration, absorption occurs rapidly and almost completely from the stomach and the upper part of the small intestine. In acidic environments the NSAIDs are highly lipophilic drugs and diffuse easily into gastric cells. As with paracetamol, rectal absorption of the NSAIDs is less predictable and incomplete although the lipid-soluble NSAIDs such as diclofenac are very well absorbed. Most NSAIDs have a relatively small volume of distribution (range 0.1–0.2 l/kg) and are all highly bound (> 90%) to albumin. Owing to the weak acidity of the NSAIDs, acidosis will increase the fraction of unionized drug, and hence diffusion from plasma into tissue. The elimination is delayed in the neonate and infant compared to adults. From the age of approximately one year, the distribution volume and elimination half-life are the same and clearance is increased compared to adults. As there is the potential for renal toxicity with NSAIDs they are not recommended for use in the first year of life because renal function is still immature in infants.

KEY LEARNING POINTS

- the effects of drugs on the body and the body's handling of drugs varies with age, maturity and severity of illness
- the young child is particularly at risk of toxic effects of single, repeated or continuous administration of analgesic drugs
- dose titration is the safest approach to analgesic administration with suitable monitoring of efficacy and adverse effects

FURTHER READING

Anand K.J.S. and Arnold J.H. (1994) Opioid tolerance and dependence in infants and children. *Critical Care Medicine* **22**, 763–767.

Anderson B.J., Woolard E.A. and Holford N.H.G. (1995) Pharmacokinetics of rectal paracetamol after major surgery in children. *Paediatric Anaesthesia* **5**, 237–242.

Berde C. (1994) Epidural analgesia in children. *Canadian Journal of Anaesthesia* **41**, 555–560.

Birmingham P.K., Tobin M.J., Henthorn T.K., Fischer D.M., Berkelhamer M., Smith F.A., Fanta K.B. and Coté C.J. (1997) 24 hours pharmacokinetics of rectal acetamonophen in children: an old drug with new recommendations. *Anesthesiology* **87**, 244–252.

Brash A.R., Hickey D.E., Graham T.P. *et al.* (1981) Pharmacokinetics of indomethacin in the neonate: relation of plasma indomethacin levels to response of the ductus arteriosus. *New England Journal of Medicine* **305**, 67–72.

Chay P.C.W., Duffy B.J. and Walker J.S. (1992) Pharmacokinetic–pharmacodynamic relationships of morphine in neonates. *Clinical Pharmacology and Therapeutic* **51**, 334–342.

Choonara I., Lawrence A., Michalkiewicz A., Bowhay A. and Ratcliffe J. (1992) Morphine metabolism in neonates and infants. *British Journal of Clinical Pharmacology* **34**, 434–437.

Eyres R.L. (1995) Local anaesthetic agents in infancy. *Paediatric Anaesthesia* **5**, 213–218.

Greeley W.J., Boyd III J,L. and Kern F.H. (1993) Pharmacokinetics of

analgesic drugs. In *Pain in Neonates* (eds Anand K.J.S. and McGrath P.J.)
pp. 107–154. Elsevier, Amsterdam.

Hopkins C.S., Underhill S. and Booker P.D. (1990)
Pharmacokinetics of paracetamol after cardiac surgery. *Archives of Disease in Childhood* **65**, 971–976.

Kart T., Christrup L.L. and Rasmussen M. (1997) Recommended use of morphine in neonates, infants and children based on a literature review. *Paediatric Anaesthesia* **7**, 5–12.

McNicol R. (1996) Paediatric regional anaesthesia: an update. *Bailliere's Clinical Anaesthesiology* **10**, 725–752.

Tucker G.T. (1994) Safety in numbers. The role of pharmacokinetics in local anesthetic toxicity. *Regional Anesthesia* **19**, 155–163.

CHAPTER 5

LOCAL AND REGIONAL ANAESTHETIC TECHNIQUES

G.A.M. Wilson, Eddie Doyle

Topical cutaneous and mucosal local anaesthesia

Instillation of local anaesthetics

Wound or dressing perfusion with local anaesthetics

Intravenous regional analgesia (Bier's block)

Infiltration analgesia

Peripheral nerve blocks

Nerve plexus blockade

Epidural local anaesthesia

Spinal (subarachnoid; intrathecal) local anaesthesia

Intrathecal opioids

Local anaesthetic toxicity: prevention, identification and management

The use of regional anaesthetic techniques in children was initially described at the turn of the century but as the safety of general anaesthesia improved, regional techniques became less common. In the last fifteen years they have enjoyed a renaissance. Regional techniques are associated with the provision of dense analgesia lasting into the post-operative period. By combining a regional analgesic technique with general anaesthesia there is a reduced requirement for volatile anaesthetic agents and opioids, with more rapid recovery and a reduction in the incidence and severity of opioid-induced side effects. An increasing concern with the humanitarian aspects of post-operative care including improved analgesia has led to increased use of regional techniques. In combination with opioids and NSAIDs, regional anaesthesia acts synergistically to produce better analgesia with a minimum of side effects. The use of various local anaesthetic techniques combined with general anaesthesia now plays a major part in the provision of good analgesia for children. Local or regional analgesia should form part of the analgesic technique for *all* paediatric patients unless there is a specific contraindication. Local and regional analgesia techniques include topical application, instillation or infiltration of the surgical field with local anaesthetic, single nerve blockade, plexus blockade and central neuraxial blockade (epidural and spinal analgesia).

Any regional anaesthetic technique should only be performed by individuals with appropriate training and experience who are aware of the potential complications of the drugs and technique to be used and who have the ability, trained assistance and resuscitation facilities to treat any potential complications. While techniques such as infiltration or digital nerve blocks and specific single nerve blocks may be performed by any doctor, more major and invasive techniques should be restricted to anaesthetists and performed under sterile conditions. Avoidable morbidity and mortality from a non-essential technique performed incorrectly is an unacceptable result of attempting to provide analgesia. Regional techniques which appear deceptively simple can be performed incorrectly and not only is the child deprived of the potential benefits of the intervention, they are also exposed to significant risks. The post-operative care of a child may have to be modified if certain regional techniques have been used and thus *appropriate* post-operative care must be provided. Regional techniques can produce a lack of sensation which may distress children if this has not been explained beforehand and presents the potential risk of injuries from incorrect positioning of a limb, pressure sores, tight plaster casts or ischaemia of muscle compartments. As with other aspects of analgesic management, education is the key.

TOPICAL CUTANEOUS AND MUCOSAL LOCAL ANAESTHESIA

The most commonly used local anaesthetic technique in children is application of a topically active local anaesthetic preparation to provide cutaneous anaesthesia for needling procedures such as venepuncture, venous cannulation and lumbar puncture. It has been shown that the main barrier to diffusion of local anaesthetic through intact skin is the stratum corneum of the epidermis which consists of layers of dead cells that have a high proportion of lipid. Amethocaine penetrates through this barrier more rapidly than lignocaine or prilocaine because it is more lipid soluble. Although EMLA cream (a 50:50 eutectic mixture of the local anaesthetics lignocaine and prilocaine) has been found to be an effective topical anaesthetic agent with a high degree of efficacy and an impressive safety profile, amethocaine has a reduced onset time and a longer duration of action than EMLA cream.

EMLA CREAM

Solid lignocaine and prilocaine mixed in equal proportions undergo a phase change to a liquid at room
temperature and this type of mixture is called a eutectic
mixture. EMLA cream consists of a eutectic mixture of
2.5% (25 mg/ml) lignocaine base and 2.5% prilocaine
base in an emulsifier. The concentration of local anaesthetic in the droplets of this emulsion is 80%. This
accounts for the efficacy of the preparation since the
effective concentration of local anaesthetic in contact
with the skin is 80% while the low overall concentration
of 5% reduces the risk of systemic toxicity after absorption. A dose of 2.5g is recommended for use in children.
A blob of cream is placed over the chosen sites and an
occlusive dressing (e.g. Opsite, Tegaderm) is applied to
ensure skin contact and to cause wetting of the stratum
corneum which speeds up absorption. EMLA cream has
been shown to be effective in relieving the pain associated with needling procedures such as venepuncture,
venous cannulation, vaccination and lumbar puncture.
EMLA cream is ineffective when used in neonates to
alleviate the pain associated with heel lancing for capillary blood sampling and has the added disadvantage of
producing capillary constriction. The minimum effective application time is one hour. It is more effective if
left in place for 90–120 minutes. The mean depth of skin
analgesia to needle insertion is highly correlated with the
duration of application and after 120 minutes exceeds
the mean skin thickness. Melanin in the skin delays
absorption. The maximal depth of analgesia to needle
insertion following application for 120 minutes has been
shown to be 5 mm and the duration of action is 30–60
minutes after removal of the cream. This suggests that
EMLA applied for two hours is likely to be more effec-

tive. When EMLA cream is used blanching of the skin at the site of application is seen in almost all subjects. This should not be considered a side effect but a predictable pharmacological effect of the compound. Both lignocaine and prilocaine have vasoconstrictor and vasodilator effects which are dependent on concentration. Constriction or blanching occurs at lower and dilatation at higher concentrations. EMLA cream has a biphasic action on the cutaneous blood vessels with a vasoconstrictive effect which is maximal after 1.5 hours followed after 2–3 hours of application by vasodilatation. The biphasic effect of EMLA cream on the cutaneous vasculature is probably the result of a slow accumulation of prilocaine and lignocaine in the dermis as they diffuse from the site of application. The initial vasoconstriction at the site of application sometimes makes venepuncture difficult (although the problem often lies at the other end of the needle!). Assays of plasma for lignocaine and prilocaine after application of EMLA to children over the age of 3 months produced maximum concentrations of 155 nanograms/ml of lignocaine and 131 nanograms/ml of prilocaine which occurred 4 hours post-application. These are both well below concentrations associated with systemic toxicity which is in the region of 6 *micro*grams/ml for these drugs. The major concern regarding the use of EMLA cream relates to the potential risk of methaemoglobinaemia. Methaemoglobin is formed by the oxidation of the ferrous iron in haemoglobin to the ferric state. It is normally formed within the red blood cell but is constantly reduced to haemoglobin by methaemoglobin reductase to maintain levels of less than 2%. Methaemoglobin has a very low oxygen carrying capacity and levels above 5% are clinically significant. Neonates and infants are particularly susceptible to methaemoglobinaemia because the iron in foetal haemoglobin (HbF) is more readily oxidized than that in haemoglobin A and infants are relatively deficient in methaemoglobin reductase. Premature babies generally have a higher methaemoglobin level than term infants and have been shown to have an increased susceptibility to acquired methaemoglobinaemia. This is the basis for the particular concern when EMLA cream is used in children aged less than one year. Two metabolites of prilocaine have been shown to cause methaemoglobinaemia – 4–hydroxy-2–methylaniline and 2–methylaniline (ortho-toluidine). Methaemoglobin levels reached a maximum of 0.85% 10 hours following the application of 5 g of EMLA cream in children aged 1–6 years. This increase has been shown to last for over 24 hours in some subjects with levels of 0.7% at 20 hours and 0.58% at 24 hours, both significantly raised compared to the control group (0.46%), leading to concerns over the possibility of accumulation with repeated applications. Application of 2 g of EMLA cream for four hours in infants less than 3 months old produced methaemoglobin concentrations ranging from 0.95 to 3.37% eight hours after application. These increases are small and unlikely to be of clinical significance unless there are repeated frequent applications or the concurrent ingestion of other inducing agents. The product is not licensed for children under 1 year of age because of these concerns but other than in the case of premature neonates undergoing repeated applications it seems that the concerns about methaemoglobinaemia associated with EMLA are not borne out by clinical problems and that recommendations which restrict its use in younger children may be unnecessarily cautious.

An alternative formulation of EMLA as a patch is available which is more convenient to use. It consists of a shallow well of EMLA in the centre of an adhesive patch. The protective front cover is removed to expose the cream and adhesive surround and this is placed on the site. The kinetics and dynamics of the EMLA patch are exactly like EMLA cream.

AMETHOCAINE

Amethocaine is more lipophilic than either lignocaine or prilocaine and thus crosses the stratum corneum barrier more easily. It is also more potent than EMLA cream. Since it is a highly lipophilic agent, amethocaine penetrates the epidermis and dermis readily and has a high affinity for neural tissue. Topical amethocaine has been shown to be at least as effective as EMLA cream in providing analgesia prior to venous cannulation. Its advantages include a more rapid onset time of 30 minutes for venepuncture in the antecubital fossa and 40 minutes for venous cannulation on the back of the hand. The duration of action after removal is about 4 hours. Like EMLA cream it must be applied under an occlusive dressing. The proprietary product is a 4% gel which was developed after much background research to establish the optimum formulation. The dosage unit is 1 g of gel (40 mg amethocaine) expressed from a 1.5 g tube. Repeat exposures to amethocaine have been shown to be safe without evidence of hypersensitivity reactions. Side effects include occasional itch in 9% of subjects and mild localized oedema in 5%. These side effects are all minor and self-limiting. Localised erythema at the site of application occurs in 37% of patients after 40 minutes (and more after longer application times) and is secondary to local vasodilatation which is a predictable pharmacological effect rather than a side effect. A study undertaken in adult volunteers in which the maximum recommended dose of amethocaine (2 g) was applied to the skin for a period of 4 hours showed measurable plasma levels of amethocaine in only 70% of volunteers. Although the toxic level of plasma amethocaine is not known, in this study levels of up to 0.2 mg/l were not associated with any adverse reactions.

An innovative amethocaine patch has also been developed, which uses a thin layer of anhydrous amethocaine gel coated onto a tinfoil central portion of an occlusive dressing. This is 'activated' by wetting the surface of the gel and then applying the patch which then behaves as the gel formulation. The attraction of this product is in its potential as an 'analgesic dressing'.

TOPICAL MUCOSAL ANAESTHESIA

There are safety implications of applying local anaesthetics to mucosal surfaces as absorption is much more rapid than through skin especially if the mucosa is inflamed. Small amounts of local anaesthetics can be applied safely to the urethra for urethral catheterization, to the perineum for cauterization of genital warts, to the site of circumcision for post-operative analgesia, under the foreskin for division of prepucial adhesions and onto the conjunctiva for analgesia after squint correction or for removal of a foreign body. The formulations available are lignocaine gel (1 or 2%) for urethral and prepucial application, EMLA cream or amethocaine gel for perineal or prepucial application and amethocaine and oxybuprocaine eye drops.

INSTILLATION OF LOCAL ANAESTHETICS

Local anaesthetics can be instilled onto small open wounds either by dropping solution onto the wound or applying a soaked dressing to the wound. Analgesia is obtained within 5–10 minutes, sufficient to allow cleaning and application of adhesive strips to close the wound. If the wound needs to be sutured, infiltration of the skin adjacent to the wound with local anaesthetic can be carried out from the cleaned, analgesed wound surface. A variety of local anaesthetic solutions can be used in this way such as plain or adrenaline containing lignocaine (1 or 2%) or bupivacaine (0.25 or 0.5%). A range of proprietary products are available, usually comprising a local anaesthetic (either lignocaine, bupivacaine, prilocaine, amethocaine or cocaine) plus a vasoconstrictor (either adrenaline, noradrenaline or octapressin). Recently a comparison of six formulations showed that bupivacaine–noradrenaline mixtures were as good as infiltration with lignocaine for suturing small lacerations in children.

Irrigation of herniorrhaphy wounds has been shown to be as effective as nerve blockade. Wound irrigation with bupivacaine for 30 seconds in children who had undergone groin surgery reduced opioid requirements in the post-operative period and resulted in a reduced incidence of nausea and vomiting compared with a control group. There was no increase in the incidence of delayed wound healing or infection.

WOUND OR DRESSING PERFUSION
WITH LOCAL ANAESTHETICS

Instillation of dilute local anaesthetics onto dressings is a useful simple method of providing analgesia for split skin graft donor sites. Bupivacaine 0.125–0.25% with adrenaline 1:400,000 up to a maximum bupivacaine dose of 2 mg/kg is placed on a foam pad which is applied to the donor site once the graft has been cut. This provides prolonged analgesia of this very painful site. To further prolong the pain relief, an epidural catheter can be placed on the surface of the foam dressing and 1–3 ml/hr of 0.125–0.25% bupivacaine via a syringe driver perfuses the dressing thereafter. This catheter perfusion system can also be used for surgical wounds and bone graft donor sites, e.g. from the iliac crest. Care must be taken not to exceed 0.5 mg/kg/hr bupivacaine (2 mg/kg/4hr).

INTRAVENOUS REGIONAL
ANALGESIA (BIER'S BLOCK)

This technique involves isolation of the forearm or lower leg with a double cuff tourniquet inflated to 20% above systolic arterial pressure and then intravenous injection of a dilute solution of the local anaesthetic prilocaine into the isolated limb. The local anaesthetic then diffuses in a retrograde fashion back up the venules and capillaries to the nerve endings in the limb. A volume of 0.4–0.8 ml/kg of prilocaine 0.5% (2.5–4 mg/kg) may be used. It is important to check that the local anaesthetic solution contains no vasoconstrictor. Venous access must be secured in the contralateral limb to allow immediate access for resuscitation. The cuff must be tested for leaks and monitored throughout with a pressure gauge as cuff failure could lead to local anaesthetic toxicity. The local anaesthetic fixes to the tissues after about 20 minutes and cuff release usually produces no adverse effects. However, on close examination and questioning some children do exhibit early clinical signs of local anaesthetic toxicity when the cuff is deflated such as circumoral tingling, light-headedness or tinnitus. Prilocaine has a proven track record of efficacy and safety. Bupivacaine should *not* be used as there have been reports of fatal cardiovascular toxicity with this technique. This technique should not be used in children with sickle cell disease.

INFILTRATION ANALGESIA

Infiltration techniques are widely used in most areas of paediatric surgery, particularly those limited to the body surface. Infiltration of closed fractures with local anaesthetic prior to reduction is possible in children (haematoma block) but may require sedation and analgesia before the injection, for example with Entonox.

Local infiltration under direct vision in the anaesthetized child is simple and is relatively free from complications. Infiltration of the wound after inguinal herniotomy is as effective as caudal analgesia or ilioinguinal nerve block. However, analgesia is limited to the skin and superficial tissues and for anything other than superficial procedures it is insufficient as the sole analgesic technique and usually requires supplementation. Possible complications include haematoma, intravascular injection and wound infection. The incidence of these complications is low and there may be a decreased incidence of side effects compared to other analgesic techniques.

For infiltration analgesia in the conscious child for superficial laceration repair and cleaning, pain and stinging on injection are common problems and lead to considerable distress. This can be minimized by applying topical local anaesthetic first as noted above, then infiltrating out from the analgesed surface. Use of small needles (27 or 29G), warming the local anaesthetic solution to body temperature and slow injection all help. Another helpful tip is to alkalinize or buffer the acidic local anaesthetic solution with bicarbonate (1 ml 8.4% bicarbonate to 10 ml 1% lignocaine). Adrenaline-free solutions must be used. The choice of local anaesthetic agent for infiltration depends on the desired duration of analgesia. Bupivacaine will produce much more prolonged analgesia and is to be preferred. The speed of onset of infiltration analgesia is comparable for lignocaine, prilocaine and bupivacaine. Maximum doses are 2 mg/kg for bupivacaine (0.8 ml/kg of 0.25%, 0.4 ml/kg of 0.5%), 3 mg/kg of lignocaine or prilocaine (0.6 ml/kg of 0.5% solution, 0.3 ml/kg of 1% solution, 0.15 ml/kg of 2% solution).

PERIPHERAL NERVE BLOCKS

DIGITAL NERVE BLOCK

This is a simple and effective technique for procedures limited to single digits. Each digit is supplied by two dorsal and two palmar/plantar nerves, which accompany the digital vessels. In the hand, 0.5–1 ml of 0.25% *plain* bupivacaine (no adrenaline) is injected on either side of the base of the digit keeping the needle at right angles to the plane of the hand. This allows both palmar and dorsal branches to be blocked. An additional small volume (0.5–1 ml) deposited over the dorsal aspect of the digit is useful for nail surgery to ensure dorsal branches of the digital nerves are blocked. A similar technique more proximally in the hand, metacarpal block, is useful if the extremity is dirty or infected and for web-space surgery such as syndactyly release. A similar technique is employed for blockade of the toes although metatarsal block may be more effective. For this the needle is introduced on the dorsal surface of the foot and directed towards the sole passing the side of the metatarsal bone in the space to be blocked. Prior to the sole being punctured, local anaesthetic is deposited as the needle is slowly withdrawn. The process is repeated on the other side of the metatarsal. Similar volumes of local anaesthetic are used. *Adrenaline should not be used* because of the risk of vasoconstriction leading to ischaemic damage. A further risk to the vascular supply arises from the compression caused by injection of too large a volume of local anaesthetic especially in the smaller child. Metatarsal/metacarpal blocks are preferable in smaller children to minimize this risk.

PENILE NERVE BLOCK

Several techniques for penile block have been described, involving either midline or lateral administration of local anaesthetic. The two dorsal penile nerves are derived from the internal pudendal nerves and innervate the dorsal surface of the penis and glans. The dorsal nerves divide into a number of branches a few millimetres distal to the pubic symphysis and this is a useful landmark for injection. In the midline technique, the pubic symphysis is identified and the needle is introduced in a caudad direction just below this point. A click may be felt as the needle penetrates Buck's fascia which encloses the neurovascular compartment. After negative aspiration, 0.5–3 ml of 0.5% plain bupivacaine are injected depending on the age of the child. *Adrenaline should not be added* to the local anaesthetic. The dorsal nerve block may be supplemented by subcutaneous infiltration of anaesthetic around the base of the penis in order to affect smaller branches which arise proximally. A study in adults undergoing circumcision under dorsal nerve block alone showed that a supplemental injection of local anaesthetic at the penoscrotal junction reduced the failure rate from 6.4% to zero. The authors suggest that this is due to the involvement of a branch of the pudendal nerve in the innervation of the ventral surface of the penis.

The lateral technique involves the injection of local anaesthetic at the '10 o'clock and 2 o'clock' positions at the base of the penis with the aim of depositing the agent closer to the two nerves which lie on either side of the vessels. In this technique, Buck's fascia is pierced from below with the depth confirmed by the needle tip striking the bone of the pubic arch. This technique is as effective as a single dorsal injection, may be easier to learn and carries less risk of puncturing dorsal penile vessels. The 'depth gauge' provided by the bony landmarks is helpful because one of the commonest reasons for failure of penile block is superficial, subcutaneous injection outwith Buck's fascia.

A subcutaneous ring block performed with 1.5–5 ml of local anaesthetic solution has been described which almost eliminates the risk of vessel injury or injection into vascular penile tissue.

Dorsal nerve block for circumcision is a simple procedure with a high success rate. Failure rates of up to 13% have been described. Duration of analgesia may be from 4 to 12 hours. Comparison with caudal block has shown a similar degree of analgesia with the benefits of a simpler technique and fewer potential complications in some studies and a shorter duration of analgesia in others. The main complications are inadvertent vascular injection or penetration or injection of the penile vascular tissue which may cause haematoma and impair perfusion of the glans. Failure of the block is usually evident immediately. Rescue analgesia with topical lignocaine gel is the quickest solution in the early recovery period, though the very distressed infant may need an opioid.

ILIOINGUINAL/ILIOHYPOGASTRIC NERVE BLOCK

This is one of the commonest techniques practised in paediatric anaesthesia and is useful for the control of pain following hernia repair and orchidopexy. The block itself is simple to perform and requires only the identification of a superficial landmark. The anterior cutaneous branch of the iliohypogastric nerve runs between the internal oblique and the transversus muscles. Just medial to the anterior superior iliac spine it pierces the internal oblique muscle to lie between it and the external oblique aponeurosis. The ilioinguinal nerve follows a similar course but pierces the internal oblique more medially. Injection of local anaesthetic deep to the external oblique aponeurosis will ensure blockade of both nerves and may also include the subcostal nerve (T12) which lies in the same plane but more cephalad.

At a point one patient-finger's breadth medial to the anterior superior iliac spine a short-bevelled 22G needle is introduced. It is usually possible to penetrate the skin and subcutaneous fat and feel the needle bounce on the aponeurosis of the external oblique muscle. As the needle rests on the aponeurosis, the weight of the syringe induces a dimpling of the surface layers. Gentle forward advancement of the needle causes the dimple to disappear as the aponeurosis is penetrated with a distinct 'pop'. Two thirds of the calculated volume of local anaesthetic (0.5–0.8 ml/kg of 0.25% bupivacaine) is then injected into the potential space between external and internal oblique. This injection should be free of resistance and a bleb is not raised if the injection is made in the correct plane. The needle is then withdrawn to the subcutaneous tissue level and redirected laterally. It is advanced down onto the bony surface of the inner aspect of the iliac crest and the remaining one third of the calculated local anaesthetic volume is deposited as the needle is slowly withdrawn to the skin. Supplementation of the block by a subcutaneous fan-like injection of local anaesthetic may enhance the effect but is not necessary. Indeed, in small infants absorption of this subcutaneous depot may result in high peak plasma concentrations of bupivacaine. For orchidopexy, incisions low in the scrotum innervated by branches from the genitofemoral nerve will not be covered and require separate local infiltration by the surgeon prior to reawakening.

Comparison of ilioinguinal–iliohypogastric block with other methods of analgesia has generally shown it to be as effective in providing post-operative analgesia as caudal and opioid analgesia. Advantages over caudal anaesthesia include avoidance of lower limb motor block while advantages over opiate analgesia include reduced nausea and vomiting. There was no difference in recovery characteristics, including time to ambulate, urinate and discharge between children given caudal blocks and those given ilioinguinal–iliohypogastric blocks. Administration of diclofenac rectally has been shown to halve the percentage of patients requiring rescue analgesia after orchidopexy. Complications of ilioinguinal–iliohypogastric block are few although there are case reports of transient quadriceps paresis following intra-operative administration of bupivacaine into the surgical field. This was ascribed to diffusion of drug through the tissues in sufficient quantities to cause a transient femoral nerve block. Misplacement of the injected local anaesthesia distally near to the inguinal ligament is quite likely to result in femoral motor block which can last for several hours and may delay discharge of older ambulant children after day case surgery. This is more likely if fanwise subcutaneous infiltration has been used, another reason for avoiding it. Deep injection directed too medially may result in a fascia iliaca block with involvement of branches of the lumbar plexus and a consequent risk of motor blockade.

INTERCOSTAL NERVE BLOCK

This provides useful analgesia following thoracoabdominal surgery, renal surgery or fractured ribs allowing earlier mobilization, better toleration of physiotherapy and an opioid sparing effect. Each intercostal nerve lies deep to the posterior intercostal membrane close to the pleura posteriorly, prior to entering the subcostal groove. It is usually easy to feel the point where the rib starts to curve anteriorly (the angle of the rib). Here the intercostal nerve is related closely to the intercostal vessels lying in or near the subcostal groove but the intercostal 'space' is quite deep at this point and is often preferred as the point of injection. The nerve continues along the lower rib margin until it gives off its anterior cutaneous branch. Throughout this portion the nerve lies between the subcostal and external intercostal muscles so that the pleura is more protected. Thus some prefer the mid-axillary line as the point of injection. Intercostal nerve block may be carried out with the patient on their side, prone or sitting up. The lateral position is preferred in smaller children taking care to extend the uppermost arm, to allow access to as many ribs as possible. After aseptic skin preparation the angle of the rib is palpated and the skin is drawn up cephalad with the palpating finger over the rib. A 22G needle is inserted perpendicular in all planes to the skin and rib until bone is contacted. The needle is then walked down the rib surface as the skin is allowed to retract, keeping the needle perpendicular in all planes to the rib until it slips off the lower edge of the rib. The needle is advanced by no more than 2 mm followed by aspiration for air or blood. If this is negative then 1–3 ml of 0.25% or 0.5% bupivacaine with 1:200,000 adrenaline is injected depending on the size of the child and the number of intercostal nerves to be blocked. This is a very vascular area and systemic uptake can be very rapid so adrenaline containing bupivacaine is preferred to increase T_{max} (time at which C_{max} is reached) and reduce C_{max} (maximum plasma concentration). A total dose of 1.5 mg/kg bupivacaine has been shown to produce safe peak plasma bupivacaine levels in both infants and neonates. Between 4 and 10 hours of analgesia may be obtained. The number and location of nerves to be blocked depends on the extent and location of the surgical wound or rib injury but usually at least an additional dermatome at each extreme of the wound must be blocked as there is considerable overlap in innervation. After each nerve is blocked, the needle tip is withdrawn to the subcutaneous tissues, the skin is retracted up onto the rib and the needle point rested on the rib surface to act as a marker for the next block performed with a fresh needle. This is because it is very easy to miss a nerve.

Intercostal nerve block may also be performed under direct vision by the surgeon at operation. An intercostal, interpleural or paravertebral catheter may be used to allow continuation of the block into the post-operative period by top-up doses or continuous infusion.

RECTUS SHEATH BLOCK

Periumbilical incisions are needed for repair of umbilical and paraumbilical hernias and for some types of laparoscopic surgery. The incision for pyloromyotomy is often also in this region. The rectus sheath encloses the rectus abdominis muscle which extends from the xiphisternum to the pubic crest and is formed by the aponeuroses of external oblique, internal oblique and transversus abdominis muscles. Although anteriorly, the sheath is interrupted by tendinous intersections, posteriorly the sheath is a continuous potential space. The rectus sheath block relies on entering this potential space at one point and depositing local anaesthetic which spreads proximally and distally. The ventral branches of the intercostal nerves T7–12 are amenable to block by this route. It is best to use a short bevelled needle and direct it perpendicular to the abdominal wall in all planes. The lateral edge of the rectus muscle is usually easy to identify by palpation and the injection point is 1 cm medial to this. The anterior wall of the sheath is identified by scratching the needle from side to side. A click indicates entry into the sheath and it then enters the rectus muscle. Further gentle advancement and scratching identifies the posterior wall of the sheath. Bupivacaine 0.2 0.5 mg/kg is then deposited after an aspiration test. A similar block carried out on the other side will ensure excellent analgesia for midline incisions.

FEMORAL NERVE BLOCK

In the pelvis the femoral nerve lies on the psoas and iliacus muscles behind the fascia iliaca. It runs parallel to the femoral vein and artery which lie anterior to the fascia iliaca. An easy mnemonic to help remember the relationships from lateral to medial is NAVEL (Nerve, Artery, Vein, Empty space, Lacunar ligament). As the vessels pass under the inguinal ligament they draw a fascial sheath with them. The femoral nerve does not lie within this sheath but lateral to it. Both the femoral nerve and vessels lie deep to the fascia lata. The presence of these fascial layers allows for the identification of the position of the blocking needle. The lateral cutaneous nerve of thigh enters the thigh deep to the fascia lata just medial and inferior to the anterior superior iliac spine. The inguinal ligament extends from the anterior superior iliac spine to the pubic tubercle and the femoral artery may be palpated inferior to the midpoint of a line drawn between these two landmarks. A 22G short-bevelled needle is introduced in a cephalad direction just below the level of the inguinal ligament. A distinct 'pop' may be felt as the fascia is penetrated. Following aspiration to exclude vessel puncture, the local anaesthetic solution is injected. A 'double pop' as the needle traverses the fascia lata then the fascia iliaca has been described. This may be too subtle a distinction especially if a short-bevelled needle is not employed. Fan-like injection of local anaesthetic solution has been described involving injection of 0.2 ml/kg of 0.5% bupivacaine one finger-breadth lateral to the femoral artery deep to the fascia. The use of adrenaline containing solutions will usually extend the duration of the block compared with plain bupivacaine.

An alternative technique involves the use of a nerve stimulator. This allows more accurate placement of the tip of the needle. In a series of 223 sciatic and femoral nerve blocks a failure rate of only 2% was found. Simultaneous blockade of the lateral cutaneous nerve of the thigh provides cutaneous analgesia to the outer aspect of the thigh. This is of particular value in plastic surgical procedures such as skin grafting where the graft is taken from the anterior and lateral aspect of the thigh.

The use of continuous femoral nerve blockade has been described as an analgesic technique to avoid the use of opioids in patients with closed head trauma. The authors used a Seldinger technique to site a 3F central venous catheter. The femoral sheath was identified by the 'double-pop' technique. A needle was inserted at right angles to the skin, approximately 1 cm lateral to the pulsation of the femoral artery just below the inguinal ligament. The double pop occurs as first the superficial fascial layer then the fascia iliaca is penetrated. A guidewire was then inserted, and a cannula advanced over it. An initial dose of 0.5 ml/kg 0.25% bupivacaine plus 1/200,000 adrenaline was administered followed by an infusion of 0.15 ml/kg/hr of 0.2% bupivacaine (0.3 mg/kg/hr). The blocks were maintained for 4–6 days in four patients with one patient requiring two supplemental doses of parenteral opioid. An alternative approach using an 18G epidural needle and a double

93

loss of resistance has also been described for continuous femoral nerve blockade. The epidural catheter was threaded 5–8 cm cephalad. A lower concentration of bupivacaine was used (0.5 ml/kg/hr of 0.125%) and was maintained for 3–5 days. In this report of the 23 children studied, only four required additional analgesia. Localized infection occurred at the insertion site in one child. Maximum plasma levels ranged from 0.67 to 0.93 micrograms/ml.

Use of a larger volume (up to 0.8 ml/kg of 0.25% bupivacaine) will result in a '3–in-1' block of the femoral and obturator nerves plus the lateral cutaneous nerve of the thigh.

NERVE PLEXUS BLOCKADE

FASCIA ILIACA COMPARTMENT BLOCK

The fascia iliaca compartment block has been described as an alternative to femoral nerve block and 'three-in-one' block for the provision of unilateral analgesia in the lower limbs. The technique has a significantly higher success rate (95%) than the 'three-in-one' block in children (20%). The fascia iliaca compartment block does not require the use of a nerve stimulator or the production of parasthesiae and is performed away from blood vessels and nerves so that the chances of inadvertent nerve injury or intravascular injection of local anaesthetic are remote. The technique involves injection of local anaesthetic solution into the fascia iliaca compartment which is a potential space between the iliacus muscle and the fascia iliaca which covers it. This space is limited anteriorly by the fascia iliaca, posteriorly by the iliacus muscle, medially by the vertebral column and upper sacrum and laterally by the inner surface of the iliac crest. Distally the fascia iliaca blends with the fascia covering sartorius and is covered by fascia lata below the inguinal ligament and so the fascia iliaca compartment extends to the lateral part of the upper thigh. The femoral, obturator and lateral cutaneous nerves traverse the fascia iliaca compartment and can be blocked by local anaesthetic solution deposited in this compartment in the thigh if a sufficient volume is injected and upward migration is encouraged by the application of distal pressure. A fascia iliaca compartment block is performed at a point 1–2 cm perpendicularly below the junction of the lateral one third and medial two thirds of the inguinal ligament. A 22G short-bevelled regional block needle is connected to a syringe of local anaesthetic solution by a length of plastic tubing and inserted perpendicular to the skin and advanced slowly until a distinct double pop is felt as it pierces first the fascia lata and then the fascia iliaca. After a negative aspiration test the local anaesthetic solution is injected while firm pressure is exerted distal to the injection site. The dose used is 2 mg/kg (0.8 ml/kg) of 0.25% bupivacaine with or without adrenaline. Plasma levels of bupivacaine with adrenaline are significantly lower than without adrenaline (median maximum plasma concentrations 0.35 (range 0.17–0.96) versus 1.1 (range 0.54–1.29) micrograms/ml).

SCIATIC NERVE BLOCK

Block of the sciatic nerve will provide anaesthesia of the anterolateral leg and the foot. If used in combination with a saphenous or femoral nerve block, anaesthesia of the leg below the knee is obtained. If the sciatic nerve is blocked at the buttock the back of the thigh is anaesthetized owing to the proximity of the posterior cutaneous nerve of the thigh. The sciatic nerve leaves the pelvis via the greater sciatic foramen lying on top of the muscles surrounding the hip joint and covered by the gluteus maximus. It then runs down in the posterior compartment of the thigh to the popliteal fossa where it divides into the common peroneal and tibial nerves. There are three principal approaches to the proximal sciatic nerve – posterior, anterior and lateral. An alternative more distal approach is to block the sciatic nerve in the popliteal fossa. Tibial and common peroneal nerve blocks have been described without information on success rates although no complications were reported in 50 patients. In the posterior approach the patient is supine with the thigh and knee flexed to 90°. The sciatic nerve lies midway between a line drawn between the greater trochanter and the ischial tuberosity. As the leg is flexed, the nerve tends to be fixed in the groove against the pelvis as it emerges from the greater sciatic foramen. Use of a nerve stimulator elicits dorsiflexion of the foot and allows safe identification of the nerve. A short-bevelled stimulating needle is introduced and is advanced while a stimulus of 1mA is produced each second. Once dorsiflexion is obtained the needle should be localized to the nerve by reducing the stimulating current to approximately 0.5 mA. The anterior approach to the sciatic nerve involves detection of loss of resistance as a large-bore needle enters the sciatic neurovascular compartment. A line is drawn from the anterior superior iliac spine to the pubic symphysis. At the junction of the middle and medial third, a line is drawn at right angles. The point at which this line intercepts a line running from the greater trochanter parallel to the inguinal ligament represents the point of needle insertion. A short-bevelled needle is used attached to a syringe. The needle is initially introduced so that it contacts the femoral shaft. It is then 'walked' medially and deeper with a constant pressure being maintained on the syringe plunger. As the sciatic neurovascular compartment is entered there is a loss of resistance similar to that felt on entering the epidural space. A dose of 0.2 ml/kg (1 mg/kg) 0.5% bupivacaine with 1/200,000 adrenaline provides rapid onset of block. In an initial study, 18 of 38 patients required no further post-operative analgesia up to 20 hours after block insertion. A failure rate of 4.8% with no complications was reported in another series of 82 cases.

BRACHIAL PLEXUS BLOCK

Nerve blocks of the upper limb are used to provide intra- and post-operative analgesia following orthopaedic and plastic surgical procedures. Upper limb blockade is usually carried out by the axillary route since this is considered to be the safest technique free of the risks of pneumothorax, phrenic nerve block and recurrent laryngeal nerve block which are associated with the supraclavicular and parascalene techniques. The axillary approach to the brachial plexus is of particular value in surgery on the hand and forearm. More proximal brachial plexus blocks will provide analgesia of the shoulder and may include areas innervated by the cervical plexus. Analgesia of the ulnar nerve distribution may, however, be less predictable. In a series of 142 brachial plexus blocks combined with intravenous sedation, carried out on 109 individuals (mean age 14.4 years) 134 were performed by the axillary route. All underwent a surgical procedure on the upper limb. A high success rate was found with only three subjects requiring supplementation of the block by the surgeon and six requiring general anaesthesia. Unsupplemented brachial plexus block will be tolerated by few children for surgery and is most useful as an adjunct to general anaesthesia to provide for peri-operative analgesia. In addition it has also been used to provide sympathetic blockade and enhance post-operative blood flow to the arm. The technique is usually contraindicated if there is a risk of a post-operative compartment syndrome. The brachial plexus emerges from between the scalenus anterior and scalenus medius muscles enclosed in a fascial sheath which continues into the distal axilla and also encloses the axillary artery. Any local anaesthetic injected into this sheath will spread proximally, increasing the likelihood of including the lateral aspects of arm innervated by the radial and musculocutaneous nerves. The arm is abducted to an angle of 90° with the forearm with the hand supinated and the elbow flexed to a right angle. This allows the axillary artery to be easily palpated against the humerus. The skin is aseptically prepared and the needle introduced into the axillary sheath at the most proximal point at which the artery can be palpated. A 'pop' may be felt as the sheath is entered, especially if a short-bevelled needle is used. After negative aspiration for blood, local anaesthetic is injected without further movement of the needle. Axillary artery transfixion should be avoided owing to the risk of haematoma. The absence of fibrous septa in the axillary sheath allows spread of local anaesthetic through the sheath and a single injection usually produces complete block. The use of a nerve stimulator confirms accurate placement of the needle before injection. The use of bupivacaine can result in good pain relief for 8–10 hours. Extension of the duration by the use of an indwelling cannula to allow subsequent top-ups has been described. The use of a radial artery catheterization set with a nerve stimulator attached to the guide wire has been described. The catheter was advanced over the wire at the point of maximal stimulation. In this case the cannula was used for intermittent local anaesthetic injections. Alternatively, for major upper arm surgery an epidural catheter may be placed in the axillary sheath by the surgeon to emerge percutaneously so that it can be used for subsequent injections or infusion of local anaesthetic solution. The brachial plexus can be blocked at a number of other points. The interscalene, parascalene and subclavian perivascular techniques have all been described. They each have a higher risk of complications than the axillary approach, including: pneumothorax; haemothorax owing to subclavian or vertebral vessel puncture or injury; inadvertent blockade of phrenic nerve, recurrent laryngeal nerve, or stellate ganglion; or inadvertent subarachnoid administration.

EPIDURAL LOCAL ANAESTHESIA

CAUDAL EPIDURAL LOCAL ANAESTHESIA

The technique of epidural analgesia using a single injection of local anaesthetic into the epidural space via the caudal approach combines the advantages of a simple technique with a high success rate and is one of the commonest local anaesthetic techniques used in paediatric anaesthesia. The technique has a wide range of indications including orchidopexy, circumcision and inguinal herniotomy as well as lower limb, pelvic orthopaedic and lower abdominal surgery. It has been used as the sole technique for inguinal hernia repair in ex-premature neonates at risk of post-operative apnoeas. Several large series describe the high success rate and low incidence of complications associated with the technique. Injection is made through the sacral hiatus which is formed by a deficiency in the neural arch of the fifth sacral vertebra covered by a ligamentous membrane known as the sacrococcygeal membrane. This is found at the apex of an equilateral triangle whose base is formed by the easily palpable posterior inferior iliac spines. A common mistake is to seek the membrane too distally and a useful cross check is to stay proximal to a line extended along the middle of the lateral aspect of the thigh with the leg flexed to 90 degrees at the hip. Under aseptic conditions a needle is advanced through the sacro-coccygeal membrane until a pop or loss of resistance is felt. It is not usually necessary to perform a formal loss of resistance technique to air or saline as is necessary with lumbar and thoracic epidural techniques. The needle should be left open for 10–20 seconds to detect venous blood or cerebrospinal fluid in the event of a venous or dural tap. Aspiration of fine epidural veins will often be negative and a period of observation with the needle open to the atmosphere is essential to detect this complication. The needle should not be advanced more than 2–3 mm into the epidural space since this increases the risk of venous puncture and dural tap. The dura normally ends at the level of the second sacral vertebra but variations in anatomy may cause it to be lower. In neonates the dura often extends to the level of the third or fourth sacral vertebra. After a negative aspiration test the selected dose of local anaesthetic solution is injected slowly. The consequences of inadvertent intravascular injection depend on the rate of rise of the plasma concentration of local anaesthetic and its maximum value. Slow, fractionated injection is safer than rapid injection of a large dose.

Bupivacaine is the local anaesthetic agent used most commonly for caudal epidural blockade because of its long duration of action. Several formulae have been described to determine dosages and volumes required to produce blockade to various levels. A formula based on the number of dermatomes to be blocked and the weight (0.06 ml/segment/kg) was shown to provide blockade to midthoracic dermatomes in 250 children aged less than 7 years, although this was using lignocaine. A simpler formula has suggested 0.5 ml/kg for sacral or lumbar blockade, 0.75 ml/kg for low thoracic blockade (T10) and 1 ml/kg for midthoracic (T8) blockade. An even simpler calculation is: for children less than 6 months use 1 ml/kg of 0.125% which will block low thoracic dermatomes, while in children above this age 1 ml/kg of 0.25% will consistently block lumbar dermatomes in children less than 20 kg, while above this weight the technique becomes inconsistent at blocking inguinal dermatomes. At all ages sacral dermatomes may be blocked reliably by 0.3 ml/kg of solution. With these smaller volumes a concentration of 0.5% will provide a longer duration of block than 0.25%. Pharmacokinetic data from several studies show that doses of 2–2.5 mg/kg of bupivacaine are associated with plasma levels of bupivacaine below 4 micrograms/ml, which normally gives concern about systemic toxicity.

Failure of the technique is usually due to inability to find the hiatus and deposit the local anaesthetic in the correct space. Although the anatomy of the sacrum is variable it is rarely so unusual that caudal injection cannot be performed by an experienced anaesthetist.

Occasionally there is no sacral hiatus present. The 'failed caudal' may be due to the use of an inadequate volume to block the required nerve roots or to undetected intravascular injection. In older children there may be unexplained failures of the technique, possibly owing to the development of fibrous septation within the epidural space, which is well described in adult patients and can result in unilateral or very restricted blocks despite appropriate volumes being injected. Local anaesthetic solution can be lost through the intervertebral foramina of the sacrum and this is seen as paramedian swelling over the body of the sacrum.

Urinary retention is less common than in the past partly because of more liberal pre-operative fasting regimens which allow fluid intake until two hours preoperatively. Varying criteria for the definition of this problem make comparisons difficult. If this potential problem is explained to the parents and child (if appropriate) as a likely consequence of the technique, its occurrence will not cause anxiety and it need not be a reason to delay discharge from hospital.

Weakness of the legs is common and may be found in 31% of subjects after 0.5% bupivacaine given to block lumbar dermatomes. It is much lower when smaller volumes of 0.5% bupivacaine are used to block sacral dermatomes only. More importantly perhaps than motor weakness is the occurrence of proprioceptive blockade in a child who is unaware of any weakness and who appears to have normal power when tested in bed but who may be unable to walk unaided. Because of this all children should be closely supervised when first walking after caudal blockade. This is much more of a real problem after caudal blockade than urinary retention and may prevent the discharge of an older child who is too big to carry. The optimal concentration of bupivacaine for caudal epidural blockade in children may be 0.125%, which has been shown to produce a block with the same duration of analgesic effect and requirements for supplementary analgesia as 0.25% but with a much lower incidence of leg weakness at one hour postoperatively, even when volumes up to 1.5 ml/kg are used. Motor blockade is less of a practical problem in young infants.

There is an incidence of venous puncture of 1.6–10.6% and this is reduced if short-bevelled rather than hypodermic needles are used. If this occurs the procedure should be restarted with an unstained needle. There are no reports of extradural haematoma after caudal epidural blockade in children. It is possible to place the tip of the needle sub-periostally and theoretically to inject into the marrow cavity of the sacrum which is equivalent to an intravenous injection, but this should be detected by a marked resistance to injection.

The incidence of dural tap is about 0.1–0.2%. Negative aspiration for cerebrospinal fluid is possible and is another reason why the needle should be left open to atmosphere after entering the space before injection of local anaesthetic when the flow of cerebrospinal fluid is usually vigorous and unmistakable. The block is usually abandoned if this occurs.

The incidence of vomiting associated with caudal epidural blockade ranges from 0 to 30%. Whether this is a consequence of caudal blockade itself or is a baseline incidence associated with general anaesthesia in children is difficult to say. Concerns about the possibility of infection mean that it is essential that this central neuraxial blockade is performed under aseptic conditions. A rare complication is an implantation dermoid owing to carriage of skin cells into the epidural space by hollow needles. Some recommend use of styletted needles or making a small nick in the skin before inserting the needle. From a large survey of over 150,000 injections, the incidence of major complications after caudal block is between 1/10,000 and 1/40,000.

CAUDAL EPIDURAL CATHETER TECHNIQUES

It is possible to insert a caudal catheter using a standard epidural kit or a caudal cannula. In infants, this allows threading of the catheter to the middermatome of the wound even when this is in the thoracic region. The epidural block can then be maintained by top-ups or continuous infusion as described below.

ADDITIVES TO CAUDAL EPIDURAL LOCAL ANAESTHETICS

Various additives to local anaesthetic solutions have been used in attempts to prolong the duration of caudal analgesia provided by a single injection. The duration of caudal blockade is usually defined as the time to the first requirement for supplementary analgesia. When plain 0.25% bupivacaine is used, the duration of block ranges from 4 to 8 hours. When plain 0.5% bupivacaine is used the duration of analgesia is up to 10 hours.

ADRENALINE

Vasoconstrictors such as adrenaline decrease the rate of vascular absorption and allow a greater mass of local anaesthetic molecules to reach the nerve membranes and increase the density and duration of the block provided. The effects of adrenaline depend on the site of injection and on the local anaesthetic used. Although it reliably prolongs the duration of blockade when used for infiltration anaesthesia and nerve blocks with all local anaesthetic agents, when used for epidural injection the effects of adrenaline tend to be less pronounced with longer acting local anaesthetics such as bupivacaine than with more hydrophilic drugs such as lignocaine. The high lipid solubility of bupivacaine causes it to be deposited in epidural fat and released slowly and the relatively short lasting actions of adrenaline tend to have little effect on prolonging its duration of action. The effect of adrenaline on the duration of action of epidural bupivacaine also depends on the concentration of bupivacaine and little effect is seen when 0.5% or 0.75% are used compared with 0.125% or 0.25%. Overall the effects of adrenaline on the duration of single shot caudal epidural block are relatively modest. Adrenaline does reduce systemic uptake and thus reduces and delays the peak plasma concentration (C_{max} is reduced and T_{max} is increased).

OPIOIDS

Several studies have provided evidence of the long lasting profound analgesia which is produced in children after the administration of caudal opioids. The median duration of analgesia after 0.1 mg/kg for lower body surgery was 12 hours (range 4–24 hours) compared with 5 hours (range 3.8–24 hours) for 1 ml/kg of 0.25% bupivacaine with 1:200,000 adrenaline and 45 minutes (range 0.3–24 hours) for 0.1 mg/kg of intravenous morphine. After penile surgery caudal morphine 0.05 mg/kg produced a mean duration of analgesia of 20 (range 10–36 hours) compared with 6 (range 4–8.5 hours) for 0.5 ml/kg of 0.25% bupivacaine. After orchidopexy, morphine 0.05 mg/kg combined with 0.75 ml/kg of 0.125% bupivacaine eliminated the need for further post-operative analgesia while over 50% of those receiving bupivacaine alone required opioid analgesia post-operatively. Assays of blood for plasma morphine concentrations after the administration of caudal epidural morphine show levels much less than those required for analgesia after systemic administration and strongly suggest that the synergistic effect of epidural opioids on analgesia is due to a local action at spinal cord level as opposed to an effect after systemic absorption. Although morphine has been used most commonly for caudal epidural application in children, the synergistic effects with local anaesthetics are also seen when other opioids such as diamorphine or fentanyl are used.

Side effects include pruritis, urinary retention, nausea and vomiting as well as hypoventilation. The most feared of these is respiratory depression. This is a well-known risk when epidural opioids are used in adults and is particularly worrying because its onset may be delayed for several hours after opioid administration, particularly if morphine is the opioid used. The largest reported series of children given caudal epidural morphine reported an incidence of 11 cases clinically important hypoventilation in 138 cases (8%). Of these 11 cases eight were aged less than 3 months and 7 received parenteral opioids in addition to caudal epidural morphine. The sensitivity of children up to the age of 3 or 4 months to opioids is well known and these results are not surprising. It is likely that a group of children aged less than three months given modest doses of opioids by any route will have a significant incidence of hypoventilation and the challenge in this group is to institute appropriate post-operative care and monitoring which will detect and treat this complication effectively.

CLONIDINE

Clonidine is an alpha$_2$ adrenergic receptor agonist. This class of drugs is widely used in medicine and anaesthesia as antihypertensives, sedatives, premedicants and analgesics. The analgesic action of clonidine when administered epidurally is probably due to stimulation of descending noradrenergic medullospinal pathways which inhibit the release of nociceptive neurotransmitters in the dorsal horn of the spinal cord. A cranial site of action may also be important. Several paediatric studies have investigated and quantified the effect of clonidine when used to supplement caudal epidural blockade produced with a local anaesthetic solution. Three groups of 15 patients undergoing subumbilical general surgical and urological procedures under general and caudal anaesthesia had caudal injections of 0.25% bupivacaine. Two groups had added to this clonidine 1 microgram/kg or adrenaline 5 micrograms/ml. The quality and duration of post-operative analgesia assessed as the time to first analgesic requirement using an objective pain score was significantly longer with clonidine (mean 16.5 hours) than with plain bupivacaine (mean 7.6 hours) or bupivacaine plus adrenaline (mean 6.3 hours). The number of children requiring no further analgesia was significantly higher with clonidine (seven subjects) than with plain bupivacaine (two subjects) or bupivacaine plus adrenaline (one subject). In a comparison of 0.25% bupivacaine 1 ml/kg with or without clonidine 2 micrograms/kg for lower limb orthopaedic surgery in 46 children, there was a significantly increased duration of post-operative analgesia in the clonidine group (mean 9.8 hours) compared with the group receiving plain bupivacaine (mean 5.2 hours) and requirements for post-operative analgesics were reduced at 12 and 24 hours in the clonidine group. The superiority of clonidine 2 micrograms/kg to adrenaline 5 micrograms/ml added to 0.25% bupivacaine 1 ml/kg for caudal use was also seen in a double blind study of 60 boys undergoing orchidopexy. The mean duration of analgesia was 5.8 hours in the group receiving clonidine compared with 3.2 hours in the group receiving adrenaline. This effect is less impressive than that seen in other studies using mixtures of bupivacaine and clonidine in children for caudal epidural use and may be explained by the fact that patients were not premedicated whereas in the previous studies sedative and analgesic premedication was used producing a synergistic effect with epidural clonidine. The addition of clonidine 2 micrograms/kg to mepivacaine 7 mg/kg for caudal epidural use in children aged 1–10 years undergoing general subumbilical surgery increased the duration of effective analgesia (as assessed by an OPS of 6) from 143 minutes to 218 minutes. Paediatric studies have found no differences between groups receiving caudal clonidine and control groups in the occurrence of significant haemodynamic or respiratory changes. Mild post-operative sedation lasted longer following caudal bupivacaine 1 ml/kg with clonidine 2 micrograms/kg (mean 9.1 hours) than plain bupivacaine (mean 5.8 hours). These times corresponded closely to duration of analgesia (9.8 hours and 5.2 hours, respectively), and this effect was attributed by the authors to superior analgesia. This study, however, used sedative premedication in all patients. The addition of adrenaline 5 micrograms/ml, ketamine 0.5 mg/kg or clonidine 2 micrograms/kg to caudal bupivacaine in unpremedicated boys produced no differences between the groups in the incidence of motor block, urinary retention or post-operative sedation. Clonidine may therefore be useful in doubling the average duration of single shot caudal epidural blocks in children at the expense of a mild degree of additional sedation. The standard intravenous formulation of clonidine (150 micrograms/ml) is preservative free but does not have a product licence for epidural administration. Clonidine alone does not provide sufficient analgesia for post-operative pain and must be added to local anaesthetics.

KETAMINE

Ketamine exerts its anaesthetic and analgesic effects by binding to a subset of glutamate receptors stimulated by the agonist N-methyl D-aspartate (NMDA) where it acts as an antagonist. These are found throughout the central nervous system including the lumbar spinal cord. Basic science research in the field of pain mechanisms has shown that as well as producing analgesia after systemic administration, ketamine exerts profound analgesic actions at spinal cord level in animal preparations. This feature, together with the minimal respiratory depressant effects of ketamine, has stimulated clinical interest in its epidural and subarachnoid administration in patients to provide post-operative analgesia. Ketamine may also have a weak effect as an agonist at opioid receptors.

Studies of caudal epidural ketamine in children have demonstrated its efficacy. In a double blind study of caudal analgesia with bupivacaine 0.25% 1 ml/kg, ketamine 0.5 mg/kg or both given after induction of general anaesthesia for inguinal herniotomy post-operative analgesia with caudal ketamine (0.5 mg/kg) was similar in quality to 1 ml/kg of bupivacaine 0.25% or a combination of the two. The duration of action of the mixture of ketamine and bupivacaine was particularly impressive with only 7% of subjects requiring any further analgesia in the first 24 hours post-operatively. This compared with 20% and 30% in the ketamine and bupivacaine groups, respectively. These results have been supported by a further study which studied a more extensive and painful procedure, orchidopexy. This study showed that ketamine 0.5 mg/kg provided a longer duration of post-operative analgesia (median duration 12.5 hours) than clonidine 2 micrograms/kg (5.8 hours) or adrenaline 5 micrograms/ml (3.2 hours) when added to bupivacaine 1 ml/kg for orchidopexy. In this double blind study of 60 boys there were no differences between groups in the incidence of urinary retention, motor block or post-operative sedation. Ketamine added to 0.25% bupivacaine therefore produces a quadrupling of the average duration of analgesia. No major sequelae have been reported after the use of epidural ketamine. It is important only to use preservative-free ketamine and to realize that there is no product licence for its epidural use. It is reassuring that animal studies have demonstrated the safety of intrathecal ketamine in a single dose with preservative and multiple doses without preservative.

LUMBAR AND THORACIC EPIDURAL LOCAL ANAESTHESIA

The use of lumbar epidural analgesia in children is not a new technique and was first described in 1954 as an alternative to general anaesthesia in high risk neonates. Epidural analgesia never became widely used in children because of difficulties in performing the technique and concerns about complications when it is performed in anaesthetized patients. It has re-emerged in recent years because of increased attention to the requirements for effective analgesia in children, realization that the post-operative course may be favourably affected by dense afferent block and the availability of appropriate well-made equipment. The introduction of small gauge epidural needles (19G) and fine epidural catheters (23G) which pass through them have made epidural analgesia feasible in the smallest of children including premature neonates. A short length paediatric Tuohy needle (18G) with an improved catheter and filter locking connector has simplified the placement and management of paediatric epidurals with fewer episodes of catheter kinkage, leakage and disconnection. In recent years single shot, intermittent and infusion epidural analgesia at the thoracic and lumbar levels have become more popular, often permitting light anaesthesia, minimal opioid use, early extubation and the avoidance of post-operative ventilation. The catabolic stress response to surgery is modified by epidural anaesthesia and analgesia and in certain circumstances there is evidence that the post-operative outcome in high risk cases is favourably influenced by epidural analgesia. Groups in which these benefits appear especially marked include patients with gastro-oesophageal reflux undergoing fundoplication and neonates undergoing repair of oesophageal atresia. Physiological differences between adults and children, namely a reduced sympathetic tone and reduced blood volume in the splanchnic circulation and lower limbs in children, result in remarkable cardiovascular stability in infants undergoing high central neuraxial blockade which in adults would cause hypotension because of sympathetic blockade.

Approaches to the epidural space in children have been described at thoracic, lumbar, sacral and caudal levels. These techniques are demanding and there is a significant failure rate particularly in smaller children. Up to the age of 6–12 months it is usually possible to cannulate the epidural space via the caudal hiatus and this avoids the potential complications of higher approaches. The sacral approach relies on the fact that the sacral vertebrae remain unfused with distinct intervertebral spaces until between 18 and 30 years of age and proponents of this approach suggest that it is both safe and that catheters are easier to keep clean than catheters placed through the caudal hiatus. Dissection of the epidural space in neonates and infants reveals that fat in the epidural space has a spongy appearance and is heavily loculated with distinct spaces between individual lobules. This is in contrast to the situation in older children and adults where lobules are more densely packed and connected by fibrous strands. This fact means that a catheter introduced into the epidural space via the sacral hiatus can often be threaded to any level in the epidural canal. The child is placed on the side and observed by a second anaesthetist and the caudal hiatus identified. After preparation of the site the epidural space is cannulated by an introducer for the catheter. This may be a Tuohy needle, an intravenous cannula, a butterfly needle, or a specifically designed blunt tipped introducer. Verification of its situation in the epidural space may be performed at this stage with a loss of resistance test to saline. The catheter is then threaded up the epidural space to a distance estimated to correspond to the appropriate nerve roots for blockade. If threading of the catheter is not entirely smooth it may indicate that the catheter has met resistance and has turned back on itself. In this case threading may be facilitated by the injection of 2–3 ml of sterile normal saline, gentle flexion and extension of the spine or partial withdrawal and reinsertion of the catheter. If these measures are unsuccessful the introducer and epidural catheter should be withdrawn and the procedure restarted. The catheter should never be advanced against resistance. Failure of the catheter to reach the desired thoracic position occurs in 15% of premature neonates and 5% of infants. Advancement of a catheter from the lumbar epidural space to the thoracic region is often tried in order to avoid performing the block in the thoracic region. In a prospective assessment of the success of this technique using a 19G catheter through an 18G needle in 39 children aged from 0 to 96 months, only 22% of catheters reached the desired level; 48% of catheters described as easily advanced remained at the L4/5 level. This suggests that the lumbar approach is not reliable for siting thoracic epidural catheters in children. A measure of the difficulties seen with epidural techniques in children is given by the fact that there were also eight difficult insertions.

Several series have described formulae to estimate the distance from the skin to the epidural space. There is a poor correlation between body weight and depth to the epidural space and wide variation with age; 1 mm/kg is a reasonable guide in infants and children above six months old. The wide variation found in the depth of the epidural space means that loss of resistance should be tested for as soon as the epidural needle has entered the supraspinous ligament. A good working rule in children between 6 months and 10 years, is to reassess the approach if the needle is further in than 1 mm/kg in case the angle of insertion is incorrect or the needle has deviated from the midline.

A single shot epidural block of up to 2 mg/kg bupiva-caine given in 2–4 fractionated doses over 5–10 minutes followed by an intravenous or subcutaneous infusion of opioid is well described as a method of providing intra- and post-operative analgesia. The use of intermittent top-ups after major abdominal, thoracic and orthopaedic surgery is a useful technique in situations where there is no high dependency unit to nurse infusions. The require-ment for opioid is reduced as is the incidence of opioid-induced side effects and there is always an anaesthetist present during the top-ups to treat any complications. For single shot or intermittent top-ups there is no reliable formula to predict the volume of local anaesthetic required and neither height, weight nor age can reliably predict the level of block after a bolus. Fractionated doses of 0.1–0.3 ml/kg for lumbar epidural top-ups and half these amounts for thoracic epidural top-ups are usually safe and effective but larger volumes may be needed if the tip of the epidural catheter is sited too low.

With infusion epidural analgesia a constant degree of analgesia can be provided. If the catheter tip is sited at the appropriate dermatomal level then low concentra-tions and volumes of local anaesthetic can be infused to produce a band of analgesia, thus minimizing the risks of toxicity and the incidence and degree of motor block. Various regimens are described for infusion epidural analgesia in children. There are no data to suggest that one is superior to others. The main concern must be to keep the total dose low to minimize the possibility of systemic toxicity particularly in neonates and small infants. Accumulation of bupivacaine occurs in neo-nates after infusions have been running for 6–12 hours because of delayed clearance and most specialist centres limit the duration of epidural infusions in neonates to around 24–36 hours.

The use of bupivacaine alone may cause problems in infants despite the provision of excellent analgesia because of the lack of sedation. This may be provided by small amounts of opioid added to the epidural solution, small doses of parenteral opioid or midazolam.

Plasma concentrations of bupivacaine during continuous epidural infusions are generally low and significantly below levels which give cause for concern. However, maximum levels in individual patients may sometimes be high. Cumulation of total and free bupivacaine is seen in neonates and cases of local anaesthetic toxicity have been reported. The minimum effective dose must be used and much lower hourly dosages should be given to neonates.

Seizures have occurred because of excessive infusion rates over many hours with cumulation of bupivacaine. Infusion of 2.5 mg/kg/hr in a one-day-old neonate after a loading dose of 6 mg/kg over 3 hours caused cardiac arrest with a plasma level of bupivacaine of 5.6 micrograms/ml. Infusion of 1.67 mg/kg/hr after 4 mg/kg over 6 hours caused convulsions in an eight-year-old child (plasma level 6.6 micrograms/ml) and an infusion of 1.67 mg/kg/hr after a bolus dose of 7.5 mg/kg over 5.5 hours also caused convulsions (plasma level 10.2 micrograms/ml). An infusion of 1.25 mg/kg/hr after a bolus of 1.25 mg/kg/hr resulted in convulsions with a plasma level of bupivacaine of 5.4 micrograms/kg.

It is known that immature nerves and nerve roots are less densely myelinated than mature ones and may be blocked by lower concentrations of local anaesthetics. It is possible to provide good analgesia in neonates with concentrations of 0.08% bupivacaine which allows infusions with less fear of accumulation. Conservative suggestions for dosages to be used for epidural infusion in children after a loading dose of 2–2.5 mg/kg of bupivacaine is to infuse a maximum of 0.2–0.25 mg/kg/hr in neonates and 0.4–0.5 mg/kg/hr in older children. In neonates and infants (in whom clearance of bupivacaine is reduced and in whom cumulation is demonstrable after 6 hours), the epidural should not be continued beyond 36 hours and these babies must be managed in an intensive care or high dependency environment. If these infusion rates are unsuccessful then the addition of a systemic or epidural opioid may be tried if it is not already included but at a much reduced dose in neonates and infants. If this is not helpful it is sensible to remove the catheter and institute an opioid based analgesic technique.

Technical problems with the equipment are common when epidural infusion analgesia is used in children. They have been prospectively audited in a large series and include obstruction of the catheter (12.7%), disconnection of the bacterial filter and the catheter (3.3%) and leakage of solution through the skin puncture site (7%). Overall the incidence of early undesired losses of epidural catheters because of these problems was 16%. Improvements in equipment design which can reduce this by 75% include better locking connections between catheter and filter and use of a paediatric length 18G Tuohy needle (50 mm) with a 21G multiple side hole closed-end catheter. Unilateral blockade is an occasional feature of epidural blockade in children with an incidence of 4% in single shot caudals, 1% in sacral blockade, 0.86% in lumbar blockade and not reported in thoracic blockade. It therefore appears to be more common with caudal approaches than more cephalad approaches and is presumably related to the presence of a dorsal median raphe (the plica mediana dorsalis) which is usually incomplete but is occasionally complete in structure and fully compartmentalizes the posterior epidural space.

Side effects include urinary retention, leg weakness, tachyphylaxis, epidural haematoma, epidural infection, and the risk of intravenous and subarachnoid injection. Use of epidural infusion or intermittent top-ups in the post-operative period requires close nursing supervision of the child. Hypotension is rarely a problem especially in children of less than eight years, but the lack of sensation may cause problems if not anticipated. Pressure sores may occur in analgesic skin unless patients are repositioned regularly and following trauma the technique is generally contraindicated because of the possibility of a compartment syndrome. Urinary retention occurred with an incidence of 11% in patients receiving epidural infusions of 0.125% bupivacaine and diamorphine and epidurals should be restricted to patients who would usually be catheterized for surgical indications. It is difficult to tease out the relative contributions to this problem of opioid and local anaesthetic but it is likely that the local anaesthetic is largely responsible because the response to naloxone is generally poor. Pruritis is seen associated with opioid and is not a problem with local anaesthetics alone. It can be managed by low doses of naloxone 1–2 micrograms/kg or ondansetron 0.1 mg/kg. An incidence of 0.45% of accidents without sequelae was found in a large retrospective survey of epidural analgesia in children. Serious complications which result in permanent neurological deficit or death are rare but are well described and have a low but definite incidence which was 1/5000 in the same survey of over

24,000 cases. Risk factors for this included multiple traumatic attempts at epidural cannulation at age less than 3 months, catheterization at the lumbar rather than caudal level and the use of the loss of resistance to air technique for identifying the epidural space. Loss of resistance to air (as opposed to saline) techniques have resulted in air emboli via the epidural veins and on occasion acute cardiorespiratory deterioration consistent with venous air embolism. This situation is worsened if there is a right to left shunt resulting a systemic air embolus and 50% of five-year-old children have a probe patent foramen ovale. The subarachnoid injection of air is also a possible risk and has resulted in temporary neurological deficit. There is experimental evidence that air in the epidural space expands if nitrous oxide is subsequently used although this effect has not been shown to be harmful. Because of these considerations most workers now recommend that a loss of resistance to saline technique should be used in preference to a loss of resistance to air technique. The loss of resistance to air technique, however, is considered by many to give a superior feel when performing epidural cannulation and has been found to result in fewer dural punctures than a loss of resistance to saline technique. The technique has the added advantage that in the event of any leakage of fluid there is no possible confusion about whether or not a dural tap has occurred. In the event of difficulty identifying the epidural space the technique should be abandoned.

Epidural abscess associated with the use of epidural analgesia for acute pain in children has not been reported. A large prospective audit of epidural analgesia in children looked at 1620 cases and found colonization of the epidural space with Candida albicans in one child who was terminally ill and who had had two sequential epidural catheters *in situ* for over 4 weeks. This child also had a necrotic epidural tumour. There is one reported superficial abscess at the insertion site of a sacral epidural catheter which did not reach the epidural canal. The experience is that with an appropriate aseptic technique for catheter insertion the use of epidural analgesia for short periods in the treatment of acute pain in children is associated with a very low rate of infection. Intravascular migration of a catheter may not be obvious because it is often impossible to aspirate blood through a 23G catheter.

Contraindications to epidural analgesia in children are similar to those in adults. Absolute contraindication include local sepsis, systemic sepsis, a coagulopathy, operator inexperience and patient or parental refusal. Relative contraindications include spinal anatomical abnormalities and neurological disease.

SPINAL (SUBARACHNOID; INTRATHECAL) LOCAL ANAESTHESIA

The commonest regional technique used unsupplemented by general anaesthesia in children is spinal (subarachnoid) anaesthesia for inguinal hernia repair in premature neonates. There is a high incidence of post-operative apnoea of about 30% in ex-premature infants undergoing general anaesthesia particularly those of less than 44 weeks post-conceptual age. This is a result of immature respiratory control mechanisms, airway obstruction, anaemia and the residual effects of anaesthetic agents. This group has a high incidence of inguinal hernia (13% in infants of less than 32 weeks at birth) and the post-operative problems that can occur may threaten life, require admission to an intensive care unit and delay hospital discharge. In a group of 36 infants undergoing spinal anaesthesia only six required supplementation of the block and there were no post-operative complications. Randomized controlled studies have demonstrated a reduced incidence of post-operative apnoea and episodes of bradycardia and hypoxaemia in this group when spinal anaesthesia rather than conventional general anaesthesia is used, although the general anaesthesia techniques could be criticized for use of 'old-fashioned' agents. Supplementation of subarachnoid blockade with sedation may be more dangerous than general anaesthesia. Apnoea can occur after unsupplemented subarachnoid anaesthesia and post-operative monitoring is required for at least 12 hours post-operatively or after the last apnoea.

Subarachnoid block is performed at the L4/5 or L5/S1 level since the end of the spinal cord lies more distal in neonates than in older infants. The child is positioned in the sitting or lateral position and restrained by a second anaesthetist during the procedure and care is taken not to obstruct the airway by overflexion of the neck as the child is positioned for the block. A sugar-coated pacifier and/or 50% nitrous oxide may be administered during performance of the block to provide analgesia. A variety of drugs and dosages have been described for subarachnoid anaesthesia in infants.

The technique of subarachnoid blockade in neonates is technically difficult and there is a significant failure rate even in experienced hands. Furthermore, even a successful block may still be inadequate for the surgical procedure which necessitates supplementation by nitrous oxide, general anaesthesia or intravenous analgesia. Traction on the spermatic cord and peritoneum during herniotomy commonly causes distress and is not covered by a spinal block. The duration of the block is relatively short and may not be sufficient for some inguinal hernia repairs. The spread of local anaesthetic solution is unpredictable and in about 12% of cases there is either very high blockade or inadequate anaesthesia. High blockade usually regresses rapidly without cardiovascular effects. The technique does not provide significant post-operative analgesia because of its short duration and some alternative method of analgesia must be provided. This may be as simple as paracetamol. Alternatively, infiltration of the wound with local anaesthetic by the surgeon (bearing in mind total dosage) or ilioinguinal nerve blockade under direct vision may be performed.

In one of the largest series of 164 ex-premature infants of post-conceptual age less than 50 weeks undergoing subarachnoid anaesthesia, 137 cases (83.5%) had subarachnoid blockade which was adequate for surgery. A further 15 (9.1%) had blockade which required supplementation by topical anaesthesia or systemic analgesia/anaesthesia. In 12 patients (7.3%) lumbar puncture could not be performed and general anaesthesia with endotracheal intubation was performed. Two patients became apnoeic during performance of the lumbar puncture and five developed a subarachnoid block so high as to produce respiratory weakness which required ventilation by either face mask or endotracheal tube. One child who received general anaesthesia developed prolonged post-operative apnoea which required ventilation. The duration of motor blockade in this group ranged from 67–600 minutes (mean 195 minutes). The remarkable cardiovascular stability which is a consistent feature of high spinal and epidural blockade in children was also seen in this series. In another large series of 140 infants where subarachnoid anaesthesia was attempted there was a 4% failure rate, repeat injection was required in 27% and supplementary sedation/analgesia was required in 7%.

Because of the limitations of spinal blockade in neonates, attempts have been made to use alternatives such as one shot caudal epidural blockade, lumbar epidural blockade, combined spinal and epidural techniques and continuous caudal epidural blockade using an epidural catheter. All of these techniques have been described in relatively few patients, although early descriptions are encouraging.

Spinal anaesthesia has also been described for controlling the stress response to surgery and is probably more effective than epidural analgesia or opioids.

INTRATHECAL OPIOIDS
(see Chapter 6)

LOCAL ANAESTHETIC TOXICITY: PREVENTION, IDENTIFICATION AND MANAGEMENT

Children are not more resistant to local anaesthetic-induced toxicity than adults. The cardiovascular manifestations of bupivacaine toxicity are of particular concern in children and present as malignant and resistant ventricular tachycardia (VT) or sudden cardiovascular collapse. In high doses bupivacaine blocks the sodium channels in the myocardium, resulting in bradycardia or re-entry tachyarrhythmias. The latter may be both enhanced or induced by a direct effect or by central autonomic stimulation. All the local anaesthetics inhibit the translocation of Ca^{2+} across the sarcolemma and the endoplasmatic reticulum. Intracellular ATP production and the sodium channel activity are also inhibited. A heart rate dependent accumulation of bupivacaine owing to kinetic differences in the blockade of sodium channels has been described. This may have important clinical implications in neonates, in whom bradycardia is poorly tolerated. Furthermore, in the neonatal myocardium the regulation of Ca^{2+} content in the cytosol is immature, and contractility as well as relaxation is more dependent on Ca^{2+} influx across the sarcolemma. Inhalational anaesthetics (halothane, isoflurane and nitrous oxide) seem to increase the risk of fatal outcome following bupivacaine-induced cardiovascular collapse in infants.

The undesired effects of local anaesthetics are determined by a number of factors including the total dose administered and the rapidity of systemic uptake. Absorption depends on the characteristics of the drug and the tissue into which it is deposited. The occurrence of local anaesthetic toxicity and its recognition have a number of features unique to the paediatric population. Poor subjective awareness owing to immaturity and concurrent anaesthesia/sedation may delay recognition of the early signs of toxicity (light-headedness, tingling, circumoral numbness, etc.). Decreased hepatic clearance and plasma protein binding and immature dermal and mucosal barriers lead to potentially increased free drug availability and cumulation, particularly in neonates and the critically ill. Children with right-to-left intracardiac shunts may be more likely to suffer local anaesthetic toxicity due to bypass of the lung first-pass uptake. Toxicity is related not only to the absolute plasma level of local anaesthetic reached but also to the rate of rise of this level, the degree of protein binding since toxicity is related to the unbound concentration of local anaesthetic agent, concurrent administration of general anaesthetics or sedatives and to increased permeability of the blood–brain barrier. The following plasma concentrations have been reported to be toxic in adults: lignocaine > 10 micrograms/ml and bupivacaine > 3–5 micrograms/ml. However, the toxicity is due to the level of free unbound drug and not to the total plasma concentration. In addition, a number of other factors influence the development of toxicity, e.g. the rise time in plasma concentration, pH, hypoxia, the concomitant use of sedatives and anaesthetics.

The new amide local anaesthetics ropivacaine and levobupivacaine produce less toxicity in adults and confirmation is awaited in children.

CNS TOXICITY

Classically there is a progression of symptoms and signs including headache, irritability, circumoral paraesthesiae, drowsiness, blurred vision and convulsions. These are rarely seen in the anaesthetized child and cardiovascular problems are usually the initial indicator of toxicity. In the post-operative period the child is generally unable to report sympions and convulsions are generally the initial event. The risk of convulsions is increased in the presence of hypoxaemia and hypercarbia. Hypercapnia decreases plasma and CSF pH, causing increased cerebral blood flow. In an acid environment local anaesthetic dissociates from plasma proteins increasing the unbound fraction. Raised cerebral blood flow will increase delivery of local anaesthetic to the brain.

CARDIOVASCULAR TOXICITY

Impulse conduction and muscle contraction are both affected by local anaesthetic blockade of Na^+ ion channels. This results in bradyarrhythmias and ectopic beats progressing to cardiovascular collapse and cardiac arrest. Bupivacaine-induced toxicity is particularly resistant to treatment causing supraventricular and ventricular tachycardias, atrioventricular heart block, premature ventricular contractions and widening of the QRS complex. Bretylium may be the most effective treatment of these dysrhythmias.

MANAGEMENT OF LOCAL ANAESTHETIC TOXICITY

Treatment should include cessation of administration, measures to ensure a clear airway, artificial ventilation with 100% oxygen and external cardiac massage if necessary (ABC of basic and advanced life support). Anticonvulsants such as benzodiazepines or thiopentone should be titrated to effect (remembering that these may also cause apnoea) and fluids, pressor agents (dobutamine) and antidysrhythmics (bretylium) given if required. Clonidine may also have a role. For the unresponsive case, extracorporeal life support should also be considered using veno-arterial bypass to support the myocardium until it recovers.

KEY LEARNING POINTS

- local or regional anaesthesia are so effective that they should form part of the pain management of all paediatric patients unless there is a specific reason not to use them

- the simplest effective technique should be used
- plexus blocks and central neuraxial blocks should only be undertaken by experienced anaesthetists
- particular care is required in neonates with technical aspects of blocks and with local anaesthetic doses

FURTHER READING

Berde C.B. (1994) Epidural analgesia in children. *Canadian Journal of Anaesthesia* **41**, 555–560.

Eyres R.L. (1995) Local anaesthetic agents in infancy. *Paediatric Anaesthesia* **5**, 213–218.

Flandin-Blety C. and Barrier G. (1995) Accidents following extradural analgesia in children. The results of a retrospective study. *Paediatric Anaesthesia* **5**, 41–46.

Freeman J.A., Doyle E., Im N.G. and Morton N.S. (1993) Topical anaesthesia of the skin: a review. *Paediatric Anaesthesia* **3**, 129–138.

McNicol R. (1996) Paediatric regional anaesthesia: an update. *Bailliere's Clinical Anaesthesiology* **10**, 725–752.

Morton N.S. (1996) Paediatric postoperative analgesia. *Current Opinion in Anaesthesiology* **9**, 309–312.

Peutrell J.M. and Hughes D.G. (1994) Combined spinal and epidural anaesthesia for inguinal hernia repair in babies. *Paediatric Anaesthesia* **4**, 221–227.

CHAPTER 6

OPIOID TECHNIQUES

Ros A. Lawson

OPIOID PHARMACOLOGY

Morphine and codeine are the two substances derived from opium that have analgesic properties. As they are naturally occurring, they are correctly termed *opiates*. All other synthetic or semi-synthetic drugs with similar effects are referred to as *opioids*. Morphine is the yardstick against which all other opioids are considered. Opioids play a major role in the management of severe pain in children but the dose must be adjusted to take account of age, maturity, severity of illness and surgical procedure. There are special requirements for neonates. The use of opioids, however administered, is a balance between satisfactory analgesia and the degree of side effects and they should usually be used in conjunction with techniques such as local anaesthesia and systemic non-opioid analgesia to minimize the opioid requirement (*opioid sparing*).

MODE OF ACTION

Opioid drugs exert their effects by binding to opioid receptors located in the brain and spinal cord (**Box 6.1**).

Opioids are also classified as agonist (produces a maximal response at a receptor), antagonist (binds to but does not stimulate the receptor and may reverse agonist effect), partial agonist (produces a submaximal response at a receptor with a 'ceiling effect') and agonist–antagonist (antagonistic at one receptor site and agonistic at another) (**Box 6.2**).

Opioid receptors	
Receptor	*Action*
Mu	Analgesia, sedation, respiratory depression, euphoria, bradycardia, pruritis, miosis, nausea and vomiting, inhibition of gut motility
Kappa	Analgesia, sedation, miosis
Delta	Analgesia
Sigma	Psychotomimetic effects (e.g. dysphoria, hallucinations), mydriasis

Box 6.1

Analgesic potency of opioids in relation to intravenous morphine

Opioid	Approximate analgesic potency versus intravenous morphine	
	Intravenous/IM	oral
sufentanil	500	–
remifentanil	100	–
fentanyl	100	–
buprenorphine	25	12.5 (sublingual)
alfentanil	20	–
hydromorphone	6.0	1.3
butorphanol	5.0	–
diamorphine	2.0	0.15
morphine	**1.0**	**0.15–0.33**
methadone	1.0	0.5
nalbuphine	1.0	–
oxymorphone	1.0	–
papaveretum	0.66	–
oxycodone	0.66	0.5–1.0
pentazocine	0.15–0.25	0.06
pethidine	0.1	0.025
codeine	0.08	0.05

Box 6.2

OPIOID AGONISTS (I.E. MU RECEPTOR AGONISTS)

Morphine is usually prepared as the sulphate salt and can be given by intramuscular, intravenous, subcutaneous, oral, rectal or spinal routes. It can be formulated as a slow-release preparation for use in chronic pain relief and in a preservative-free form for epidural or intra-thecal use. When administered orally, morphine is well absorbed from the gastrointestinal tract but is subject to 'first-pass metabolism'. This means that a significant proportion of the drug is metabolized by the liver and gut wall and excreted in the bile, thereby decreasing the actual amount of drug delivered to the systemic circulation (bioavailability is decreased). In practice, this means that a much larger dose of drug is required when given by the oral route. Morphine is primarily metabolized in the liver to morphine-3-glucuronide and morphine-6-glucuronide. This second metabolite is twice as potent as morphine itself as an analgesic and has a much longer half-life. In renal impairment it is the accumulation of morphine-6-glucuronide that causes the prolonged opioid effect as this metabolite relies on renal excretion. The clearance of morphine-6-glucuronide may be reduced by the non-steroidal anti-inflammatory drugs which may partly explain the synergism between these groups of drugs. Only 10% of actual morphine is excreted by the kidneys. Morphine-3-glucuronide is anti-analgesic and produces central nervous system stimulation which may be seen in infants as 'morphine jerks' or in older children as muscle spasms, especially after orthopaedic surgery.

Pethidine (meperidine) is used infrequently in children but may be useful as an alternative drug for patient-controlled analgesia in selected cases. It was the first synthetic opioid developed and is approximately 10 times less potent than morphine. It can be administered by all conventional routes although giving pethidine subcutaneously is reported to be excessively painful. Metabolism occurs mainly in the liver where the primary metabolite is norpethidine. Norpethidine has a very long half-life (15–20 hours) and as well as having mu agonist activity, it also has non-opioid central nervous system excitatory effects. Norpethidine toxicity can result in twitching, tremors and potentially convulsions. It is only likely to occur when relatively high doses are used or when excretion is impaired such as in renal disease.

Papaveretum is a semi-synthetic mixture of opium derivatives of which 50% is morphine. It has been used effectively as an infusion in infants but has no great advantages over morphine.

Diamorphine is rapidly hydrolysed to morphine. It is more lipid soluble than morphine and may therefore penetrate the blood–brain barrier or dura more easily, making it popular for epidural or intrathecal administration. It can be reconstituted in a wide variety of concentrations which makes it particularly useful for subcutaneous administration and for use in terminal care.

Fentanyl is a synthetic opioid with a potency 60–80 times that of morphine. Its extreme lipid solubility means it has a rapid onset but shorter duration of action. There are no active metabolites. These features mean it is used extensively as an intravenous intraoperative analgesic and also in combination with local anaesthetic drugs in the epidural space. Its elimination half-life is prolonged after high doses and prolonged infusion. Newer preparations such as the fentanyl lollipop ('Oralet': oral transmucosal fentanyl citrate) and the fentanyl patch (fentanyl transdermal system) have recently been developed.

Alfentanil is a synthetic opioid with one fifth to one third the potency of fentanyl. Alfentanil is less lipid soluble than fentanyl or sufentanil. It has a quick onset of action reaching a peak effect in 60–120 seconds and has a short duration of action after a single dose owing to a low distribution volume and fast clearance. It is very useful for short painful procedures and can be used along with propofol to facilitate tracheal intubation without muscle relaxants. After prolonged infusion, its half-life gets longer the longer it is infused (prolonged context-sensitive half-life). Like the other opioids, alfentanil is mainly eliminated via the liver. In premature babies and neonates the clearance of alfentanil is low and the half-life is considerably prolonged. When infused as the sole agent in ventilated babies, alfentanil produces chest wall rigidity which interferes with ventilation.

Sufentanil is a synthetic opioid which is 5–10 times as potent as fentanyl. It is more lipid soluble than fentanyl and therefore has a rapid uptake into well-perfused tissues and a rapid onset of action. It is highly protein bound and clearance is primarily by hepatic metabolism. It can be used as an intravenous bolus or infusion or epidurally alone or in combination with local anaesthetics.

Remifentanil is a mu agonist which is metabolized by blood and tissue esterases which results in a very short half-life which is independent of dose, duration of dosing and of hepatic or renal clearance. Its context sensitive half-life is constant at about 3 minutes however long it is infused. It has a very rapid onset of action and has an analgesic potency about 100 times that of morphine. It may find a place as a 'stress response controller' for major surgery, for neonatal anaesthesia and for paediatric cardiac anaesthesia. The possibility of an acute opioid withdrawal state occurring after prolonged infusion cannot be excluded.

Codeine is the other naturally occurring opiate and is effective when given intramuscularly or orally for mild to moderate pain. It is metabolized in the liver and 10% of the original dose becomes morphine. Codeine must never be given intravenously as catastrophic hypotension may result. *Dihydrocodeine* is related to and is an alternative to codeine. *Oxycodone* has similar properties and indications. *Hydrocodone* is another opioid with a similar half-life to codeine and is used in oral preparations.

These four drugs are often manufactured in combination with a non-opioid analgesic such as paracetamol. This will sometimes limit the total dose of opioid that can be given as the maximum daily dose of paracetamol is limited.

Methadone is a long-standing synthetic opioid mostly used in the management of chronic pain in children. It has a much longer half-life and consequently a much longer duration of action than the other opioid drugs used. It can be used to wean patients from prolonged opioid therapy (>1 week) as may occur in intensive care patients. It can be given orally or intravenously.

Hydromorphone is a derivative of morphine and can be used orally, rectally and parenterally in children. It is occasionally useful if an alternative opioid is required for a PCA regime.

Tramadol is a weak opioid with a potency comparable to that of pethidine. It can be used orally or parenterally in children with negligible respiratory depressant effects. The analgesia obtained is often insufficient for severe pain and there is a high incidence of emesis and a significant incidence of dysphoria. Some patients feel better with tramadol than when other opioids are used.

THE USE OF OPIOIDS IN NEONATES

The fact that neonates feel pain and require pain relief is now undisputed and reflected in the change in practice over recent years with more anaesthetists prescribing and using opioids after major neonatal surgery. The problem has always been concern regarding the increased sensitivity of the neonate to serious side effects of opioid drugs such as respiratory depression. There are a number of reasons why this should occur. The neonate has proportionately more of its cardiac output distributed to the vessel-rich tissues of the brain and also has an immature blood–brain barrier. Thus any opioid given will have a more profound effect than that in an older infant. The very young infant has an immature ventilatory drive. Opioids also take longer to be metabolized in the neonate and have a lower clearance. It has been shown that a fourfold reduction in the elimination half-life of morphine takes place within the first four years of life. Furthermore, there is marked inter-patient variability, particularly in the neonate and even more so in the preterm baby. Pharmacodynamic sensitivity should not, however, preclude the neonate from receiving opioid analgesia provided there is adequate monitoring in the correct setting and facilities are available for immediate correction of any complications (**Box 6.3**). This usually means in practice a neonatal intensive care unit with equipment for intubation and ventilation on hand. It is particularly important to consider the use of adjuvant techniques such as regional anaesthesia in neonatal pain relief to minimize the opioid requirement.

Opioid safety

- patient selection
- safe prescribing
- safe preparation
- monitoring the patient for efficacy and adverse effects
- monitoring the delivery equipment

Box 6.3

SAFE USE AND MONITORING OF
OPIOIDS IN CHILDREN

The level of monitoring required for children and infants receiving opioid drugs is essentially the same regardless of the routes by which they are administered. It is paramount that all staff are familiar with current protocols. The first stage in safe use of opioids in children is appropriate selection of the patient and tailoring the drug, dose and route of administration to that particular patient. Individual protocols, drug regimes and treatment of side effects should be designed for each route of administration (see **Appendices 2, 4, 8, 9**).

PRESCRIPTION

All drug prescriptions should be written on order sheets plus the drug prescription chart and care taken to ensure these are legible and specific. There have been a number of recently reported situations where unclear or misleading prescriptions have led to inaccurate and sometimes dangerous doses of opioids being given. Often it is the difference between milligrams and micrograms that is unclear and it is recommended that these words should be written out in full. The position or configuration of the decimal point in a prescription is another common source of confusion and hospital policy needs to be specific about how this is addressed. Writing the dose in words and figures is a useful safety measure analagous to writing a bank cheque! Prescriptions should include initial plans for 'breakthrough' or 'rescue' analgesia and provision for the treatment of side effects (see below). The name or contact number of the person who is to be called if there are problems also needs to be included on the order sheets. This is most likely to be the acute pain team nurse or the duty anaesthetist (see **Appendices 2, 4, 8, 9**). Measures to avoid double prescription of opioids by different routes must be rigorous

PREPARATION

When the initial syringe of opioid is prepared for infusion or bolus administration, the drug concentration and diluting fluid used should be clearly labelled with the label attached so as not to obscure syringe gradations. It is also helpful to label any connecting tubing to avoid confusion with other drugs being given. The dose of opioid drug being added to diluent should be checked by two members of appropriately trained and assessed staff. A patient check using name band and prescription charts is essential. Pre-filled opioid syringes can be obtained commercially or can be manufactured by the local pharmacy. These contain a standard drug concentration (e.g. morphine 1 mg/ml) which eliminates dilution errors but potentially can lead to errors in pump programming. Many paediatric units standardize the morphine dilution for body weight with a maximum concentration of 1 mg/ml. The most commonly used formula is:

Morphine sulphate 1 mg/kg in 50ml. of 5% dextrose or 0.9% saline (= 20 micrograms/kg/ml) 1 ml/hr = 20 micrograms/kg/hr

MONITORING

Monitoring of children receiving opioids comprises regularly checking the efficacy of analgesia, actively looking for adverse effects and double checking the equipment being used to deliver analgesia. If these observations are made hourly, this allows closer titration of the technique to the child's requirements. Any child receiving opioid drugs should be nursed in a part of the ward where they are easily visible and monitors can be observed. A high dependency level of care is usually appropriate with a minimum staffing ratio of 1 nurse to 4 patients. Neonates should be managed in an intensive care environment with 1:1 nurse to patient ratio.

PATIENT MONITORING

Monitoring of the efficacy of analgesia is with an hourly pain assessment. In older children, a simple four-point self-report scale is sensitive enough provided it is used when the child is moving as well as when at rest (e.g. $0 =$ no pain; $1 =$ mild pain; $2 =$ moderate pain; $3 =$ severe pain). A nurse assessment using the same scale is appropriate in younger children or in those who cannot indicate their level of discomfort. More complex pain assessment tools may be used but are often too impractical for hourly use (see Chapter 3). The most important adverse effects of opioids are respiratory depression, excessive sedation, nausea and vomiting, ileus, urinary retention and itching. Several studies have shown that respiratory rate is a late and insensitive indicator of opioid overdosage and does not correlate accurately with oxygen saturation. It has been shown that assessment of oxygen saturation by pulse oximetry whilst the child is breathing air is the best and least invasive way of detecting early respiratory depression. Thus continuous oximetry is recommended at least for the first 24 hours along with hourly recordings of the saturation and respiratory rate. When respiratory rate is recorded, it should be with the child at rest and unstimulated. The continuous oximetry can perhaps be modified if the child is clinically well and beginning to ambulate or move around. Sedation levels need to be documented hourly to assess oversedation or inappropriate sleep pattern. This can be done using a simple four-point scoring system (0 = spontaneous eye opening; 1 = eyes open to verbal stimulus; 2 = eyes open to gentle shaking; 3 = unrousable). Oxygen saturation readings in children breathing air will be above 94% in most cases which is an acceptable level of arterial oxygen tension (10 kPa = 75 mm Hg). As the child becomes oversedated with an opioid, the arterial and alveolar CO_2 tension increase owing to inadequate ventilation. This means that the arterial and alveolar O_2 tension falls with consequent decrease in oxygen saturation. Build up of CO_2 will also cause a deepening level of sedation. However, if the child is breathing supplemental oxygen, the arterial CO_2 can rise to very high values before the oxygen saturation falls. This explains why the pulse oximeter will be a less sensitive monitor in situations where oxygen therapy is being used. In these cases, more intensive observation of sedation levels will be required. Some episodes of desaturation may be explained by underventilation owing to excessive pain or to a painful procedure. Hourly recordings of nausea and or vomiting and other side effects are documented using a simple score (0 = none; 1 = nausea only; 2 = vomiting × 1 in last hour; 3 = vomiting × >1 in last hour) (see **Appendices 2, 4, 8, 9**).

EQUIPMENT MONITORING

Hourly recordings of the residual volume of the infusion syringe should be made and a check of the pump position, settings and function. The integrity of the syringe and extension tubing and its connections should be checked hourly, looking in particular for leaks, cracks and loose connections. The docking of the syringe in the pump should also be checked to ensure that the syringe barrel is correctly immobilized and the syringe plunger is correctly gripped and is moving appropriately. The pump should be mounted horizontally no more than 80 cm above the patient's heart level. There should be an anti-free flow (anti-siphonage) valve in place in all infusions and, for concurrent administration of opioids and intravenous fluids through the same cannula, an anti-reflux valve should be incorporated in the infusion line. The infusion site should be checked hourly for leakage, extravasation, inflammation or occlusion.

A standard monitoring protocol and chart are very helpful (see appendix for examples). It is important, however, that monitoring is linked to action to improve analgesia if it is inadequate and to treat adverse effects if they are detected.

ADVERSE EFFECTS AND THEIR MANAGEMENT

The effectiveness of opioids may be limited by the incidence and severity of adverse effects. The incidence is more or less the same for equianalgesic doses of different drugs, although individual patients may feel better with one particular drug than another. Opioid-related adverse effects can be minimized by use of opioid-sparing techniques (local/regional analgesia, NSAIDs and or paracetamol) and by careful titration of the dose hourly (**Box 6.4**).

Respiratory depression and sedation

Opioids can cause this potentially fatal and much feared complication by depressing the central respiratory drive and also causing a partially obstructed upper airway due to oversedation. It will be compounded by the use of any

---

Adverse effects of opioids

- respiratory depression
- sedation
- alteration of sleep pattern
- nausea and vomiting
- slowing of gut motility
- constipation
- urinary retention
- itching
- histamine release
- muscle spasms
- pupillary constriction (miosis)

Box 6.4

other drugs causing sedation and these include antihistamines and some anti-emetics, e.g. phenothiazines. It is more likely in the very young child or infant, in those with organ failure owing to accumulation of morphine or active metabolites, in those with an abnormal airway and in those with respiratory or neuromuscular disease. In addition, if a local anaesthetic technique is being used, which becomes more effective at a particular time, then an opioid will have a relatively greater effect (e.g. when an epidural is topped up with local anaesthetic). Opioids should not be given concurrently by different routes as their sedative and respiratory depressant effects will be compounded. Respiratory depression happens rarely but is the main reason why meticulous attention needs to be paid to the monitoring of children receiving these drugs as discussed above. If a child is noted to be oversedated, have a consistent pulse oximetry reading of less than 94% or a respiratory rate of less than 20 breaths per minute in an infant or less than 12 breaths per minute in an older child, then there is opioid overdosage until proved otherwise. All patients receiving opioids in whatever form should have oxygen, suction, face mask, self-inflating bag and the opioid antagonist naloxone available immediately. Initial management consists of ensuring airway patency, administering oxygen and discontinuing any opioid drug being given. If the respiratory depression is severe, e.g. the patient is cyanosed and/or bradycardic, then naloxone should be given IV immediately by the ward nurses. An initial dose of 2–4 micrograms/kg should be given and repeated to a total of 10 micrograms/kg. The action of naloxone is shorter than most opioids and a continuous infusion of 10 micrograms/kg/hr may be required to maintain reversal. If no venous access is available the naloxone can be given via an intraosseous needle in the same doses as for intravenous administration or intramuscularly at a higher dose of 10–100 micrograms/kg. The on-call anaesthetist should be notified and any additional respiratory or circulatory support commenced. In severe overdosage, especially in a baby, ventilatory support may be required. Any precipitating factors should be sought such as concomitant use of sedative drugs. Checks should be carried out on the infusion equipment to exclude pump malfunction. Once the initial problem has been rectified, it is likely that opioid administration should cease for some time to enable blood levels to decrease before recommencing the infusion at a lower rate.

Nausea and vomiting

This is thought to be caused by opioid stimulation of the chemoreceptor trigger zone in the medulla of the brain and can be a particular problem in the older child, after upper abdominal or renal surgery and in those with a past history of post-operative emesis or motion sickness. Moderate or severe pain is also a potent cause of nausea and vomiting especially if the pain has a visceral origin. It is often dose related and the first line in management may be to reduce the dose of drug given. Some anti-emetics can cause extra-pyramidal signs in children if given frequently, e.g. metoclopramide and prochlorperazine. It is unwise to prescribe these drugs regularly. The 5–HT3 antagonist drug ondansetron has been efficacious in several studies and does not produce sedative or extrapyramidal problems. Transdermal hyoscine has also been used to good effect as there is often a component of motion sickness to opioid-induced nausea. Giving a premedicant drug such as trimeprazine in low dose (e.g. 1–2 mg/kg) appears to reduce the incidence of PONV. Low dose droperidol is another alternative (**Box 6.5**). Sometimes changing to a different opioid will decrease the incidence of nausea and vomiting in a particular patient.

▼ Anti-emetic drugs

- ondansetron 0.1 mg/kg iv, 8–12 hourly; or 0.1 mg/kg orally, 8–12 hourly
- prochlorperazine 0.1 mg/kg orally as syrup (1 mg/ml); or 0.15 mg/kg rectally as suppository (5 or 25 mg), 8–12 hourly
- trimeprazine 1 mg/kg orally
- transdermal hyoscine
- cyclizine 1 mg/kg iv or orally, 8–12 hourly
- droperidol 1–10 micrograms/kg, 12 hourly

Box 6.5

Itching

The cause of the pruritus induced by opioids is unclear. It is more common when spinal opioids are used. It is usually generalized but often manifests as an itchy nose. It should be distinguished from a localized histamine release occasionally seen at the site of injection. Antihistamine drugs are often tried to decrease symptoms but care needs to be used in case they increase the level of sedation. Chlorpheniramine is most often used at a dose of 0.1 mg/kg but should not be used in infants. It may be safer to use a small dose of naloxone which does not affect the analgesic properties of the opioid especially if pruritis is associated with epidural or spinal opioids. A bolus dose of 0.5 micrograms/kg can be given and repeated every 15 minutes up to three times or a low dose infusion at 1–2 micrograms/kg/hr can be started. Analgesia will not be diminished in most cases by these low doses. Ondansetron, 0.1 mg/kg may be effective in reducing pruritus caused by epidural or spinal opioids. These latter two techniques have the tremendous safety advantage of *no additional sedation*.

Urinary retention and gastrointestinal symptoms

The side effects of urinary retention, gut immotility and constipation may also respond to a low dose of naloxone, 0.5–2 micrograms/kg. In small babies, gentle suprapubic pressure will allow bladder emptying but it may be necessary to catheterize a patient with troublesome urinary retention as the discomfort from a full bladder may be worse than the original pain. Prophylactic urinary catheterization is recommended by many who use epidural or spinal opioids, for major surgery and where a lumbo-sacral local anaesthetic block is to be used. Postoperative ileus may be exacerbated by opioids whatever the route of administration but the patient groups who are at risk will often have contraindications to laxatives or suppositories. The problem can be minimized by using opioid sparing techniques. Laxatives, suppositories and micro-enemas may be required in severe cases.

Muscle spasms

Skeletal muscle spasm may be seen as chest wall rigidity (particularly when the potent fentanyl analogues are used) or more commonly as adductor muscle spasms in orthopaedic patients receiving parenteral morphine after surgery. This may be due to the cumulation of stimulatory metabolites such as morphine-3–glucuronide. Morphine sparing co-analgesia with NSAIDs and paracetamol is very helpful and regular low dose diazepam, 0.1 mg/kg orally up to 6 hourly is very effective but may cause some additional sedation.

INTRAVENOUS TECHNIQUES

INTERMITTENT INTRAVENOUS ADMINISTRATION

An intravenous opioid given as a bolus dose is the best way to achieve rapid analgesia with satisfactory analgesic levels often achieved within 5–10 minutes depending on the lipid solubility of the opioid used. However, as with any intermittently administered drug, fluctuating blood levels with resultant variable analgesic levels will occur. The concept of the 'analgesic corridor' demonstrates the effect of giving an IV bolus of drug intermittently (**Figure 6.1**). In addition, the time taken for the drug to exert true central nervous system effects with potential side effects or complications may be greater than the

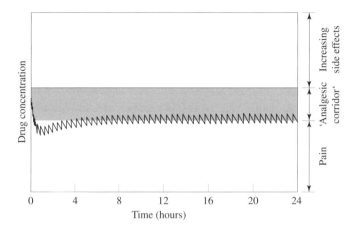

Figure 6.1
**Patient-controlled analgesia is more likely to maintain blood
concentrations of the drug within the 'analgesic corridor'**

initial time to analgesic effect. This has implications for
monitoring. Thus this technique is useful in the peri-
operative and recovery room setting and may also be of
use in the accident and emergency department provided
staff are aware of the level of monitoring required. The
regular use of intermittent bolus doses of IV opioids is
impractical on a busy ward but may be considered as a
'low tech' solution for an individual patient where the
nursing ratio is very poor but where there is no suitable
infusion equipment or in the emergency field setting.

Using the principle of titration, small repeated bolus
doses of morphine can be used and titrated to clinical
effect. In children greater than 3 months of age, an
initial 'loading' dose of 100 micrograms/kg can be given
slowly over 3–5 minutes and a 10 minute interval
allowed before reassessing the need for further analgesia. No more than three boluses within 2 hours are
recommended. Thereafter, morphine can be given as a

bolus of 50–100 micrograms/kg over 5 minutes, every 3 hours if appropriate. In children between 1 and 3 months of age, an initial loading dose of 50 micrograms/kg can be given slowly over 3–5 minutes and a 10 minute interval allowed before reassessing the need for further analgesia. In infants less than 1 month of age an initial dose of 5 micrograms/kg is advised with careful reassessment before further increments are administered up to a total of 25 micrograms/kg.

For the recovery room management of children who have had loading doses of opioids, titration with smaller bolus doses given every 5 minutes is very useful. The doses are comparable to the programme settings for PCA (20 micrograms/kg, 5 minute interval).

Often it will be more satisfactory to convert to a continuous infusion regime (see below) after the initial loading dose has achieved therapeutic effect (see **Figure 6.1**).

Fentanyl is often used in the day surgery setting to provide rapid initial analgesia with a short duration of action usually in combination with another form of analgesia such as NSAID or local block. The penalty, however, is a higher incidence of nausea and vomiting. It is also useful in the recovery room as an opioid with rapid effect to 'tide the child over' until a more suitable method of post-operative analgesia is employed or as a method of providing 'breakthrough analgesia'. In term infants greater than 1 month of age, a loading dose of 0.5 micrograms/kg can be used, waiting at least 2 minutes before giving any further boluses. A maximum of 6 doses is recommended in a 2 hour period. Chest wall rigidity is a possible adverse effect.

IV methadone has been used as a method of providing prolonged post-operative pain relief in paediatrics. This can be titrated with a loading dose of 0.1–0.2 mg/kg followed by 0.05 mg/kg increments every 10–15 minutes until analgesia is achieved. This can last for up to 12 hours after which a further dose of methadone can be given over 20 minutes.

CONTINUOUS INTRAVENOUS INFUSION

The use of a continuous infusion of opioid will provide a more consistent and constant level of analgesia as the 'peak and trough' situation of bolus dosing is avoided. However, each infusion will still require titration to the needs of the individual patient. In paediatric practice it is often an excellent method of pain relief in infants and younger children unable to use patient-controlled analgesia. The dosage regimes will depend on age and whether the child is to be ventilated or not. In children greater than 1 month of age, morphine infusions of between 10 and 30 micrograms/kg/hr provide adequate analgesia with an acceptable level of side effects. At these rates, no impairment of ventilation was found in 44 patients recovering from cardiac surgery with a minimal analgesic blood level of 12 ng/ml, less than that previously measured in adult studies. Morphine clearance in term infants greater than 3 months of age is comparable to children from 1 to 17 years old. In neonates age 1–7 days the clearance of morphine is one third that of older infants and elimination half-life approximately 1.7 times and so infusion rates should be reduced to around 4 micrograms/kg/hr. Morphine is the opioid most frequently used and studied but papaveretum has also been used as an infusion in infants between 1 and 6 months to good effect (**Box 6.6**).

Ideally there should be a dedicated intravenous cannula and connection to the infusion using an anti-free

▼ **Intravenous morphine infusion regimen**

- Morphine 1 mg/kg in 50 mls 0.9% saline (≡0.02 mg/kg/ml, i.e. 20 micrograms/kg/ml); maximum 50 mg in 50 ml
- Age 0–1 m: up to 0.004 mg/kg/hr, i.e. 4 micrograms/kg/hr ≡ 0.2 ml/hr
- >1–3 m: up to 0.010 mg/kg/hr, i.e. 10 micrograms/kg/hr ≡ 0.5 ml/hr
- >3 m: up to 0.020 mg/kg/hr, i.e. 20 micrograms/kg/hr ≡ 1 ml/hr
- (may need up to 40 micrograms/kg/hr ≡ 2 ml/hr)

Box 6.6

flow valve (anti-siphon valve). If a concurrent opioid infusion has to be given through the same cannula as intravenous fluids, it should be connected via an anti-reflux valve. Syringes should be made up in a concentration and volume designed to minimize the need for frequent changes and also allow a reasonable volume of drug to be delivered so that dead space and infusion pump innacuracy do not become significant.

Problems with use of continuous infusions arise from misconceptions about the time it takes to achieve an increase or decrease in blood levels. As the half-life of morphine is at least 3 hours in the older child and considerably longer in the neonate, altering the rate of infusion will not have a significant effect for several hours depending on the length of time the infusion has been running for. This may be as long as *five* half-lives. Thus inadequate analgesia should be treated by a bolus as directed above. If undesirable side effects are a problem, then the infusion needs to be discontinued until these have resolved before resuming at a lower dose, usually about 50% lower than the previous dose.

PATIENT-CONTROLLED ANALGESIA

Patient-controlled analgesia has been shown to be safe and effective in children as young as age 5 years and compares favourably with continuous morphine infusion in the older child. The child self-titrates to a level of analgesia that is satisfactory to them and is associated with the minimum severity of adverse effects. PCA allows for variation in the opioid requirement between patients and in the same patient over time. The child has control over their own analgesia which has considerable psychological benefits. It also allows the child the chance to anticipate painful procedures such as physiotherapy. There is also a 'built in' safety net as the child can only self-administer the drug when their sedation level allows it. This safety net only works when the patient is the sole 'button-presser'. If a well-meaning relative or untrained member of staff administers a bolus from the pump when the child has not indicated a requirement, then the patient is taken out of the PCA safety loop and the child may receive excessive drug. The PCA pump is programmed to give a small bolus of opioid from the syringe when the hand-held button is pushed by the child. The pump can be programmed in several ways:

- Bolus only (with a predetermined lockout time during which no further opioid can be received)
- bolus dose plus continuous background infusion
- continuous infusion only

PATIENT SELECTION

Any child who understands the basic concept of PCA and can operate the demand button is suitable. Children from age 5 years can operate the device but should be assessed on an individual basis. Mentally handicapped children or those with physical disabilities or injuries to the hands may not be suitable. The hand-operated demand buttons can be adapted to allow activation by pressure pads placed under the elbow, knee or by an air pressure switch operated by blowing into a tube. PCA opioid administration is applicable after most major surgical procedures, in sickle cell disease and in the management of some children with chronic pain.

CONTRAINDICATIONS

Any situation in which the use of opioid is contraindicated such as raised intracranial pressure or upper airway abnormality precludes the use of PCA. The only other contraindications are patient unwillingness or lack of ability to use the machine.

PATIENT AND PARENT PREPARATION

The efficacy with which PCA will be used depends on prior education of the patient and it is important to visit pre-operatively and show the pump and button to be pressed. Parents often voice concern regarding the possibility of their child overdosing themselves on opioid. The inherent safety aspect of the technique therefore needs to be explained (see **Appendices 3, 4**).

EQUIPMENT

- suitably sized, easily identified patient activation button which is easy to use and bleeps on being pressed. Alternative designs for patients unable to press a button should be available.
- ease and flexibility of programming to encompass a wide range of patient weights (bolus dose in micrograms or mg or preferably in micrograms/kg; lock-

out interval of 1 minute and above; background infusion optional and programmable in micrograms/kg/hr)

- standard syringe size or prefilled cartridge to minimize dilution errors
- compact, durable, lightweight, mains/battery operated
- lockable key pad and syringe holder
- clear visible display of stored data; memory capacity should be capable of holding at least 24 hours worth of data
- standard interface for data retrieval, storage, processing and generation of hard copy
- comprehensive alarm functions for mains/battery failure, occlusion, overdelivery, empty syringe, programming errors

Ideally the pump should be attached to a dedicated peripheral cannula. In practice, the cannula is also used for a concurrent IV infusion, in which case non-return and anti-free flow valves should be used to prevent free flow of opioid into the patient and prevent reflux of drug up concurrent infusion lines.

LOADING DOSE

An initial bolus dose of opioid is usually required before commencement of PCA so that therapeutic levels of analgesia are achieved quickly (see intravenous bolus opioids). This can be programmed into the pump setting but in children it may be easier to give an appropriate loading dose separately and omit the loading dose from the PCA pump programming.

BOLUS DOSE

This is the amount of drug that will be given when the PCA button is pressed. Morphine is the drug that is usually used in paediatric practice. It has been found that a bolus of 20 micrograms/kg of morphine provides a reasonable starting bolus dose in most patients. As with all regimens there may be considerable patient variability in opioid requirement and thus the bolus dose may need to be adjusted once the level of analgesia has been evaluated. The bolus dose needs to be that which provides maximal analgesia with the minimum of side effects and this will be easier to determine once several sets of pain and side effect scores have been done.

DOSE DURATION

Usually this is programmed as 'stat' on the pump, which means the bolus dose will be given at a rapid rate. However, occasionally a child may complain of stinging at the IV site which may be relieved by a slower rate of administration which can be incorporated into the pump settings (e.g. over 5 minutes). Stat delivery may also result in a pressure surge in the IV line which includes anti-free flow and anti-reflux valves as these require an opening pressure to be reached before forward flow occurs. The occlusion alarm in many PCA pumps is set to be activated at 100 mm Hg and this threshold may have to be raised to 150 mm Hg to prevent false occlusion alarms.

LOCKOUT TIME

This is the time interval during which no further opioid can be given by the pump. It is really the main safety feature of the machine and lasts from the end of the last dose for the pre-programmed number of minutes. The time will depend on the pharmacokinetics of the drug being used and usually with morphine ranges from 5 to 10 minutes. This allows time for both the analgesic and side effects of a bolus dose to be felt before another dose can be given. If analgesia appears to be inadequate it should be the bolus dose that is increased rather than the lockout time decreased in the first instance. If side effects are a problem, it may be that the lockout time needs increasing.

BACKGROUND INFUSION

We have found that the use of a background infusion usually for the first post-operative night provides improved analgesia and sleep pattern. A low dose rate of 4 micrograms/kg/hr is effective. The background infusion should be discontinued if the patient is excessively sedated. When PCA is starting to be weaned, it is usually the background infusion that is discontinued first.

DRUG PREPARATION

In general, morphine is the opioid of choice and should be prepared in such a concentration that a minimum volume of 0.5 ml is given with each bolus and there is no need for a frequent change of syringe, thus minimizing the risk of drug preparation errors. Fentanyl, pethidine (care with norpethidine toxicity), nalbuphine, hydromorphone, piritramid and tramadol have also been used in paediatric PCA sometimes in cases where morphine has given unacceptable side effects (**Box 6.**7).

OTHER ROUTES OF PCA ADMINISTRATION

The subcutaneous and epidural routes can be used in children. With subcutaneous PCA, the feedback from

---

PCA pump settings

- PCA pumps should be programmed only by members of the pain team qualified to do so
- The pump programme should only be accessible using a key supervised by this team
- Recommended drug concentration is morphine 1 mg/kg in 50 ml 0.9% saline (= 0.02 mg/kg = 20 micrograms/kg/ml); max 50 mg in 50 ml
- Bolus dose 0.02 mg/kg, i.e. 20 micrograms/kg = 1 ml; max bolus dose = 1 mg
- Lockout time 5 minutes
- Background infusion 0.004 mg/kg/hr, i.e. 4 micrograms/kg/hr = 0.2 ml/hr (especially in the first 24 hr)

Box 6.7

the site of injection may allow the child to learn to time the bolus doses better and use the device more effectively. Conversely, in some children, discomfort felt at the time of injection may deter the child from using the PCA as often as required.

NURSE OR PARENT-CONTROLLED ANALGESIA

The range of patients receiving opioids in an individually controlled manner can be increased if a nurse or parent is allowed to press the demand button within strictly set guidelines (**Box 6.8**). This would include children less than 5 years of age and those mentally and physically unable to push the demand button themselves. Monitoring for such patients has to be at least as intensive as that for conventional PCA. Most regimes for NCA utilize a higher level of background infusion (up to 20 micrograms/kg/hr) with a longer lockout time of

---

**Guidelines for nurse or parent
controlled PCA**

- Pump activation
    - pain score 2 or more (quite or very sore)
    - patient request
- Contraindications to pump activation
    - pain score 1 or less (asleep or not really sore)
    - sedation score 4 (unrousable)
    - respiratory rate less than 12 breaths per minute in a child greater than age 5 or less than 20 breaths per minute in a child under 5 years of age
    - Oxygen saturation less than 94% breathing air

Box 6.8

around 30 minutes. Another option, for example, for neonates, would be a small bolus dose with no background infusion (5 micrograms/kg with a lockout time of 20 minutes). This should not decrease the safety of the technique as long as strict protocols are adhered to.

MONITORING

The basic guidelines for monitoring and safe use in children receiving opioids by any route should be adhered to as above.

PUMP FUNCTION

Regular checks on the pump settings, power supply and residual volume in the syringe are essential to ensure correct pump function. Hourly recordings of the number and proportion of valid demands (i.e. those that result in drug delivery) will allow assessment of the child's usage of the pump and whether adjustments need to be made to the programme. Assessing number of demands may indicate that the child is using the button inappropriately and further tuition or encouragement may be required. The patency of tubing and cannula needs to be checked to ensure continued delivery of the drug

INADEQUATE ANALGESIA

Pain scores consistently greater than 2 indicate the child is receiving inadequate analgesia. This may be due to incorrect usage of the device which can be rectified by increased supervision. However, it may be that there has been an error in programming, drug dose or pump malfunction and this needs to be checked if the child continues to experience pain.

ADVERSE EFFECTS

The adverse effects of opioids given via a PCA pump are no different from any other route and should be managed as indicated on pages 139–144. Sometimes an adverse effect such as nausea will deter the child from pressing the button and this should be managed promptly to ensure that an appropriate level of analgesia can be maintained.

WEANING FROM PCA

This should be individualized and is achieved when pain scores are satisfactory and the number of demands for a bolus decreases. If a background infusion has been used it is usually best to discontinue this first and then consider increasing the lockout time. It may be appropriate to leave a pump connected even if the child appears not to be using it. Sometimes the psychological benefits may require a little longer weaning time or the continued analgesic requirements may have been misjudged.

SUBCUTANEOUS TECHNIQUES

In appropriately selected cases, the subcutaneous route of administration is a useful alternative. A subcutaneous cannula may be sited in the conscious child under topical local anaesthetic cream cover or while the child is anaesthetized. A 24G cannula can be inserted easily into the subcutaneous tissue of the anterior abdominal wall or the deltoid area of the upper outer arm and secured with adhesive tape or a transparent dressing. An infusion pump can be connected using a spiral-type connector to allow greater mobility and less tension on the cannula site. It is a particularly convenient route of administration in orthopaedics because these children often require parenteral analgesia for up to 72 hours but wish to eat and drink and mobilize. Morphine sulphate or diamorphine are most often used by the subcutaneous route. The volume of the injection and infusion should be small (maximum 1 ml) and the first one or two injections via the cannula may sting and cause some redness or itching at the site. If this is severe, check that the cannula has not been inadvertently placed *intradermally* rather than subcutaneously. A slow rate of injection or infusion helps to minimize injection pain.

It is important to recognize that there are certain clinical situations where the use of the subcutaneous route may be unwise or contraindicated. These are situations such as the hypovolaemic child or one in which there may be significant fluid compartment shifts post-operatively such as major intra-abdominal surgery or extensive burns. In situations such as these, a depot of opioid may form at a subcutaneous site of inadequate perfusion and then when perfusion improves, the child is at risk of receiving a substantial bolus dose of the drug resulting in adverse and potentially dangerous side effects.

INTERMITTENT SUBCUTANEOUS BOLUS

The subcutaneous bolus route can be convenient for nurse-administered rescue analgesia or as part of a 'low-tech' protocol for on-demand analgesia. The pharmacokinetics and dynamics are similar to the intravenous route provided peripheral tissue perfusion is stable and adequate.

CONTINUOUS SUBCUTANEOUS INFUSION

Subcutaneous infusions of morphine can be used to good effect in younger children and those unable to use a PCA machine (**Box 6.9**).

INTRAMUSCULAR ADMINISTRATION

There is now little place for the intermittent, as-required intramuscular injection in paediatric pain management. Intramuscular injections are frequently feared by children who will often suffer operation-induced pain rather than ask for another injection of analgesia. A solution is to

---

▼**Subcutaneous morphine infusion regimen**

- Morphine 1 mg/kg in 20 ml 0.9% saline ($\equiv$0.05 mg/kg/ml, i.e. 50 micrograms/kg/ml); maximum 50 mg in 20 ml
- Age 0–1 m: up to 0.005 mg/kg/hr, i.e. 5 micrograms/kg/hr $\equiv$ 0.1 ml/hr
- >1–3 m: up to 0.010 mg/kg/hr, i.e. 10 micrograms/kg/hr $\equiv$ 0.2 ml/hr
- >3 m: up to 0.020 mg/kg/hr, i.e. 20 micrograms/kg/hr $\equiv$ 0.4 ml/hr [may need up to 0.6 ml/hr]

Box 6.9

place an intramuscular cannula while the child is anaesthetized or under topical local anaesthesia and this is then managed as for a subcutaneous cannula. This is a low tech way of dealing with analgesia on demand where infusion pumps are not available (**Box 6.10**).

Intramuscular codeine phosphate can be given perioperatively (1 mg/kg) in cases where deep sedation is to be avoided such as upper airway surgery or neurosurgery. It is useful for mild to moderate pain and can cause respiratory depression in very small babies or where other opioids or sedatives are being given. Codeine should never be administered by the intravenous route as catastrophic hypotension may result.

ORAL ADMINISTRATION

Oral preparations of opioids are less commonly used in the management of acute pain but are of occasional use

---

'On-demand' analgesia with morphine via a subcutaneous or intramuscular cannula

- draw up an ampoule of morphine sulphate, 10 mg/ml and dilute to 10 ml with 0.9% saline
- draw up calculated bolus dose from this 1 mg/ml solution
- <1 m = 25 micrograms/kg = 0.025 ml/kg (use 1 ml syringe)
- 1 m–3 m = 50 micrograms/kg = 0.05 ml/kg (use 1 ml syringe)
- >3 m = 100 micrograms/kg = 0.1 ml/kg (use 1 ml syringe up to 10 kg)
- dilute with 0.9% saline to 1 ml total volume if <10 kg
- inject via cannula
- flush cannula with 0.5 ml of 0.9% saline
- repeat on demand up to every 2 hours
- monitor as for IV infusion

Box 6.10

as an interim method before using simple oral analgesics. They are often manufactured in combination with NSAIDs or paracetamol. Oral administration results in presystemic elimination by liver metabolism (first-pass effect) and sometimes the side effects of these metabolites may be undesirable. The amount of drug reaching the systemic circulation and thus the opioid receptors after first pass metabolism is termed the bioavailability of the drug. Codeine is the most commonly used oral opioid. Enteral bioavailability is around 50–60%, analgesia being reached in around 20 minutes and peaking at 60–120 minutes after an oral dose. Recommended doses are 0.5–1 mg/kg every 6 hours. Codeine elixir comes as a preparation of 15 mg in 15 ml and the tablets as 15 mg, 30 mg and 60 mg. Oral morphine is often administered as a syrup, more commonly in the setting of chronic pain management (**Box 6.11**). The combination of a slow-release morphine preparation with morphine syrup for breakthrough pain is used to good effect.

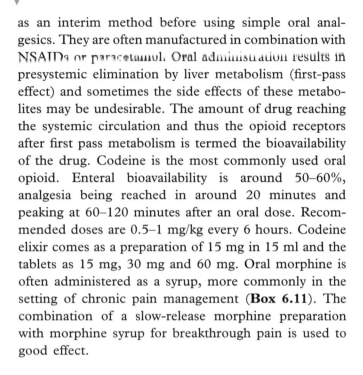

Morphine oral preparations (oral dose is approximately 3 times the IV dose)

- syrup: 1 mg/ml
- drops: 20 mg/ml
- tablets 30 mg
- tablets, sustained release: 15, 30 and 60 mg

Box 6.11

TRANSMUCOSAL ADMINISTRATION

Less traditional routes of administration of opioids are of interest in paediatric pain relief and oral transmucosal fentanyl citrate has been manufactured as a sweetened lozenge or lollipop for the child to suck. This preparation is of particular use as premedication or when a sedative technique is being used, although it must be ensured that standard monitoring policies are being followed as for all opioids. Its use has been associated with a decrease in respiratory rate and oxygen saturation and can cause nausea and vomiting. The usual dose for children is 5–10 micrograms/kg and it is supplied in doses of 200, 300 and 400 micrograms. It is not recommended for use in children under 15 kg.

TRANSDERMAL ADMINISTRATION

Fentanyl has also been manufactured in a patch formulation for transdermal application. However, its pharmacokinetics are unsuited for use in post-operative pain relief. Fentanyl patches have found some application in the management of chronic pain in older children and the usual monitoring precautions should apply.

RECTAL ADMINISTRATION

This route is used infrequently in paediatric practice and should be used with care owing to the great inter-patient variability in bioavailability and absorption. When morphine is given rectally, the bioavailability is reported to be similar to an oral dose if administered in solution. However, there may be a much greater variability in absorption if given in a solid rectal form. This is emphasized by at least one reported fatality in an infant receiving rectal morphine suppositories.

EPIDURAL AND INTRATHECAL ANALGESIA

The injection of opioids into the epidural or intrathecal space allows action on the spinal cord opioid receptors situated in the substantia gelatinosa region of the dorsal column of the spinal cord. Several studies have shown the technique to have useful application in paediatric post-operative analgesia. The procedure is most likely to be performed by an anaesthetist peri-operatively and subsequent administration of drug through a catheter should also be supervised by members of the anaesthetic team. More rarely, during spinal surgery a surgeon can inject or place a catheter in the epidural space under direct vision at the end of surgery.

ANATOMY
The epidural space is a potential space around the dura in the cranium extending to the sacrum. In children it can be approached directly via the thoracic or, more commonly, lumbar vertebrae or via the sacral hiatus into the caudal epidural space. Its contents differ from the adult in that there is more loose areolar tissue as well as fat, connective tissue and blood vessels – which may favour a more longitudinal spread of a particular drug. The intrathecal space is usually reached by performing a

lumbar puncture. The primary site of action of a drug is at the spinal cord regardless of the means of approach. Spinal opioids exert their analgesia effects by reducing neurotransmitter release at the presynaptic level, and by hyperpolarizing the membrane of dorsal horn neurons at the post-synaptic level. An opioid introduced into the epidural space passes through the dura, arachnoid membrane, cerebrospinal fluid and reaches the opioid receptors (mu 1 and 2, kappa) in the spinal cord. The drug also enters the systemic circulation via the epidural veins and is distributed to the epidural fat.

DRUGS USED

The use of opioids in the epidural space has the advantage of providing analgesia without the sympathetic or motor blockade seen when local anaesthetics are used, although these side effects may not be seen in children to the same degree as they are in adults. Morphine is the most frequently used and studied drug in both adults and children, although fentanyl and diamorphine are also effective. It is the lipid solubility of the drug which determines how it behaves in the spinal cord. Lipid solubility affects the dose required, the speed of onset, the duration of action and the degree of complications. If a drug has greater lipid solubility, there will be a more rapid transfer across the dura to the opioid receptor sites and therefore a quicker onset of analgesia. However, the duration of action is also shorter as the drug will be removed more quickly from receptor sites by blood flow. Morphine has a relatively low lipid solubility compared to, for example, fentanyl. This means that it may take longer to act but also stays for a greater length of time in the CSF. This has implications with regard to spread of the drug to a site rostral from the point of injection (i.e. the drug will be carried by the CSF circulation upwards towards the brain). The analgesic effect of less lipid-soluble opioids is less dependent on the dermatomal site of injection. Morphine stays longer in the CSF which means it is more likely to spread cranially and cause unwanted side effects such as respiratory depression. It is important to realize that this side effect may not manifest until up to 24 hours after the initial injection. Rostral spread of a drug will also account for other side effects such as nausea, itching and urinary retention. The well-documented risk of delayed respiratory depression means that strict monitoring guidelines need to be instituted before epidural or intrathecal opioids are used in paediatric practice and for this reason many centres only utilize this means of analgesia in a high dependency setting. If a more lipid-soluble drug such as fentanyl is used, a greater proportion of the dose is absorbed systemically and a dose similar to that given systemically is required. Fentanyl is therefore often best used in combination with a local anaesthetic drug in an infusion technique and the combination of opioid and local anaesthetic is well known to produce synergistic effects.

Clinically, the objectives of coadministering epidural opioids with subanaesthetic concentrations of local anaesthetics are important as reduction in the dose of both drugs is achieved, enhancement of the degree of pain relief is seen and there is a reduction in the incidence of adverse effects produced by both opioids and/ or local anaesthetics.

EPIDURAL ADMINISTRATION OF OPIOIDS

Opioids can be administered into the epidural space either as a bolus dose or continuous infusion. Bolus doses can be either a single shot, usually at the start of surgery, or intermittently via a catheter placed in the epidural space. The bolus can consist of a single opioid – usually morphine or an opioid/local anaesthetic combination. If a continuous infusion is used to administer the opioid, there is always some local anaesthetic drug added to the infusion. One study has shown that the analgesia obtained by a single bolus of morphine is comparable to a continuous infusion of fentanyl and local anaesthetic, although with the infusion the incidence of nausea and itching was less. If a child is getting local anaesthetic only through the epidural catheter, a small dose of fentanyl (0.5–1 micrograms/kg) given epidurally and flushed with saline may 'smooth' the analgesic effect where the local anaesthetic did not give complete analgesia. A problem arises where a child has received spinal opioids but does not appear to have adequate pain relief. Ideally another non-opioid analgesic such as a NSAID can be effective but it may be that parenteral opioids will be required. If this is the case, the patient should be intensively monitored until the effects of the spinal opioid are judged to have worn off as there is a high risk of respiratory depression with concurrent administration of opioids by different routes.

PRESCRIPTIONS FOR ADMINISTRATION OF EPIDURAL OPIOIDS

All prescriptions for the epidural opioid bolus or infusion should be clearly written on a standardized epidural chart as well as the same prescription on the drug chart (**Box 6.12**). In addition, it should be documented clearly that the patient should *not be prescribed any other form of opioid or drug with sedative properties* unless authorized by the pain team. Management strategies for the treatment of breakthrough pain and the treatment of side effects need to be prescribed and a contact number available in case of problems.

MONITORING

Basic monitoring standards need to be followed as in the general guidelines. The main difference in patients receiving spinal opioids is the complication of delayed respiratory depression. However, it is important to recognize that ventilatory impairment can occur at *any* time after opioid administration and a high degree of vigilance is required. Early respiratory depression is more likely to be caused by fentanyl whereas later problems occur owing to rostral spread of morphine. The time interval from injection is unpredictable (e.g. 3.5–24 hours) and has an increased incidence in children under 1 year of age. Nevertheless, it has also been reported in the older child. It is more likely with a higher dose of spinal opioid and also if opioids have been used peri-operatively. Respiratory depression is thought to be a risk until 24 hours after the last administration of spinal

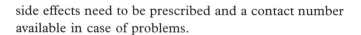

Recommended regimens for epidural opioids

- add preservative free morphine 500 micrograms to 50 mls of 0.125% bupivacaine (i.e. 10 micrograms per ml), *run at 0.1–0.4 ml/kg/h* (not in neonates) [≡1–4 micrograms/kg/h morphine]
  or
- add fentanyl 100 micrograms to 50 mls of 0.125% bupivacaine (i.e. 2 micrograms per ml) (not in neonates) *run at 0.1–0.4 ml/kg/h*

Box 6.12

opioid therefore the child should never receive this method of analgesia as a day case.

INTRATHECAL ADMINISTRATION OF OPIOIDS

Intrathecal opioids are usually given as a single dose at the time of lumbar puncture. Spinal catheters have been used in adults but there is little experience with their use in children and associated technical difficulties with the small catheter may be prohibitive. Morphine is given as a single dose of 0.02 micrograms/kg and compares favourably to PCA with no increase of serious side effects.

GUIDELINES FOR MANAGEMENT ON WARD/HDU

All patients should have a patent IV cannula in place for 4 hours after the last dose of fentanyl and for 12 hours after the last dose of morphine. Oxygen, naloxone (with appropriate dose documented and readily available) and suction must be immediately available at the bedside. Continuous pulse oximetry with alarms set to a lower limit of 94% should be used. Hourly documentation of pain and sedation scores is recommended. Regular checks on the epidural site to look for any leakage or inflammation are also important. The level of block should be checked regularly if epidural local anaes-thetics are also being used. It is essential that all ward staff differentiate between those children receiving local anaesthetics only and those in whom opioids have been added to an epidural regimen.

ADVERSE EFFECTS

As well as the respiratory depression discussed above, the other side effects noted with opioids have a signifi-cant incidence when the drugs are used epidurally or intrathecally. The micturition reflex is inhibited in up to 30% of children. Naloxone 0.5–2 micrograms/kg and a low dose naloxone infusion is very effective while analgesia is maintained. Catheterization is often needed and many anaesthetists will do this prophylactically in any child receiving epidural or intrathecal opioids. Nausea and vomiting may occur in 40% of children and is treated with anti-emetics as above. Itching occurs in 40–50% and is treated with low dose naloxone or ondansetron.

KEY LEARNING POINTS

- opioids can be used safely and effectively in children of all ages
- titration, assessment and monitoring are essential for safety
- intermittent intramuscular opioids should not be used in children unless absolutely necessary in which case use an im cannula

FURTHER READING

Bray R.J., Woodhams A.M., Vallis C.J., Kelly P.J. and Ward-Platt M.P. (1996) A double-blind comparison of morphine infusion and patient controlled analgesia in children. *Paediatric Anaesthesia* **6**, 121–127.

Doyle E., Harper I. and Morton N.S. (1993) Patient controlled analgesia with low dose background infusions after lower abdominal surgery in children. *British Journal of Anaesthesia* **71**, 818–822.

Doyle E., Mottart K.J., Marshall C. and Morton N.S. (1994) Comparison of different bolus doses of morphine for patient controlled analgesia in children. *British Journal of Anaesthesia* **72**, 160–163.

Gillespie J.A. and Morton N.S. (1992) Patient controlled analgesia for children; a review. *Paediatric Anaesthesia* **2**, 51–59.

Hartley R. and Levene M.I. (1995) Opioid pharmacology in the newborn. *Bailliere's Clinical Paediatrics* **3**, 467–493.

Howard R.F. (1996) Planning for pain relief. *Bailliere's Clinical Anaesthesiology* **10**, 657–675.

McIntyre P.E. and Ready L.B. (1996) Acute pain management – a practical guide. WB Saunders, London.

Morton N.S. (1993) Development of a monitoring protocol for safe use of opioids in children. *Paediatric Anaesthesia* **3**, 179–184.

Thompson J.P. and Rowbotham D.J. (1996) Remifentanil – an opioid for the 21st century. *British Journal of Anaesthesia* **76**, 341–343.

CHAPTER 7

NON-OPIOID ANALGESIC TECHNIQUES

Kay O'Brien

Non-steroidal anti-inflammatory drugs (NSAIDs)

Paracetamol

Nitrous oxide

NON-STEROIDAL ANTI-INFLAMMATORY DRUGS (NSAIDs)

Previously, the main indications for using NSAIDs included the treatment of childhood rheumatic disease and other chronic inflammatory conditions, closure of the patent ductus arteriosus and symptomatic treatment of pyrexia or musculoskeletal pain. NSAIDs are becoming increasingly important in the treatment of mild or moderate acute pain in children. The NSAIDs may be used as the sole method of pain relief, or in combination with a local or regional nerve block, particularly in day case surgery. NSAIDs are often used in combination with, or to facilitate weaning from opioid analgesia. While the 'opioid sparing' effect of NSAIDs is not yet quantified in children, it is likely to be around 30%, as reported for adults. There appears to be little difference between the analgesic efficacy of the different NSAIDs, although only 50–60% of children will respond to a given NSAID. Most are given orally or rectally, although some, e.g. ketorolac or tenoxicam, can be given by injection. There are differences between the NSAIDs, most notably in their anti-inflammatory effect which provides a basis for the clinical classification used in **Box 7.1**. It is important to realize that very few of these drugs have official product licences for treating paediatric acute pain but a large literature and widespread adoption by clinicians support their use.

MECHANISM OF ACTION

The anti-inflammatory effect of NSAIDs is thought to be due to inhibition of prostaglandin biosynthesis. This

Classification of NSAIDs		
Antiflammatory effect	Drug group	Example
Weak	Acetaminophen	Paracetamol
Mild to moderate	Propionic acid derivatives	Fenbufen Ibuprofen Ketoprofen
	Fenamic acid derivatives	Mefenamic acid
	Non-acidic drug	Nambumetone
Strong	Salicylic acid derivatives	Acetylsalicylic acid Trisalicylate Choline magnesium trisalicylate
	Pyrazolone derivatives	Oxyphenbutazone Phenylbutazone
	Acetic acid derivatives	Diclofenac Indomethacin Sulindac
	Oxicam derivatives	Piroxicam Tenoxicam

Box 7.1

occurs via inhibition of the enzyme cyclooxygenase which is necessary for the conversion of arachidonic acid to stable prostaglandins. During the inflammatory process prostaglandin is produced locally and disruption of this process leads to a reduction in inflammation. This effect of NSAIDs appears to be dose related, with good analgesic and anti-pyretic effects at low doses and anti-inflammatory actions at higher doses. NSAIDs also have other effects on cellular function. Their ability to affect protein–protein interactions in the cell membrane leads to inhibition of superoxide anion generation, and chemotaxis of phagocytes. Activation of neutrophils is also affected and this action may be one of the primary mechanisms of action of NSAIDs. Platelet function is also inhibited by NSAIDs. Thromboxane B2, which promotes platelet aggregation, is a product of prostaglandin biosynthesis, and therefore its levels are decreased by NSAIDs. Bleeding time is prolonged by all NSAIDs except the non-acetylated salicylates as they only weakly inhibit platelet prostaglandin biosynthesis. Aspirin, unlike the other NSAIDs, irreversibly acetylates and inactivates prostaglandin synthetase so bleeding time returns to normal only when new platelets are released into the circulation.

Pharmacokinetics

While the specific pharmacokinetic actions of each NSAID may vary, general properties can be attributed to the various drugs. All non-steroidal anti-inflammatory drugs are weak organic acids that can be rapidly and almost completely absorbed orally. Following oral ingestion peak plasma concentrations are normally achieved within 2–3 hours. However, newer preparations may include enteric coating or slow release coating to further delay absorption. NSAIDs have a small distribution volume as they are highly bound to plasma proteins, especially albumin. Consequently patients with low albumin levels have increased free fractions of the drug available which influences both metabolism and elimination. They are either oxidized primarily in the liver by cytochrome P-450 or conjugated by glucuronide. Renal excretion accounts for less than 10% of the unmetabolized drug, but in patients with renal compromise toxic metabolites may accumulate. Other less important modes of excretion include biliary excretion and enterohepatic recirculation. For age-related differences, see **Table 7.1**.

DOSAGE

Suggested doses and duration of therapy vary according to each drug, each approved route of administration and each country. Paediatric usage is extremely variable as licensing of the different NSAIDs varies from country to country, e.g. ketorolac is widely used in the US while diclofenac is the more commonly used NSAID in Europe. Reference should be made to the appropriate product information sheet. (See **Table 7.2**.)

Table 7.1 Age-related differences in elimination half-lives of NSAIDs (in hours)

	Premature babies	Mature babies	1–7 y	7–15 y	Adults
diclofenac	–	–	1.3	–	1.1
indomethacin	20.7	14.7	8.5	–	7.1
naproxen	–	–	–	12.0	14.0
piroxicam	–	–	–	35.0	55.0

Table 7.2 NSAID dosing

NSAID	Number of doses (mg/kg) per day	Maximum daily dose (mg/kg/day)
diclofenac	1 × 3	3
ibuprofen	10 × 4	40
indometacin	1 × 3	3
ketorolac	0.5 × 4	2
naproxen	7.5 × 2	15
piroxicam	0.4 × 1	0.4

PROPIONIC ACID DERIVATIVES

Ibuprofen has an antipyretic effect in children at a dose of 5–10 mg/kg and has an anti-inflammatory effect similar to high dose aspirin therapy. The anti-inflammatory dose is 30–40 mg/kg/day in 3–4 divided doses (maximum dose 2400 mg). Severe reactions including haemolytic anaemia and pure white cell aplasia have been reported. Ibuprofen is available as a non-prescription drug in many countries.

ACETIC ACID DERIVATIVES

Diclofenac sodium is a phenylacetic acid derivative used extensively in Europe. Standard oral tablets, dispersible tablets and enteric coated tablets are available. The parenteral (intramuscular) formulation is not very suitable for children because of injection pain and the high incidence of residual pain at the injection site. In paediatrics, suppositories of 12.5 mg, 25 mg, 50 mg and 100 mg are most often used and are well absorbed in 30–60 minutes. The dose is 1 mg/kg up to 8 hourly. It is good practice to discuss the use of suppositories with parents and child in advance and to gain verbal consent for their use. They should not be used without consent.

Another useful formulation of diclofenac is as topical eyedrops which give effective analgesia after squint correction in children.

Ketorolac tromethamine is available as an intravenous injection, tablets and eyedrops. It has been widely used in paediatrics as an intravenous dose of 0.5 mg/kg which is based on paediatric pharmacokinetic data. The initial adult dose currently recommended is 0.15 mg/kg with subsequent titration to effect.

In the neonate, indomethacin has been used to induce closure of the patent ductus arteriosus. Indomethacin is an acetic acid derivative with potent antipyretic and anti-inflammatory effects but is associated with a high incidence of serious side effects, such as gastrointestinal bleeding and hepatitis. It is not suitable for the management of acute pain in children.

SALICYLATES

The salicylates include aspirin, choline magnesium trisalicylate and choline salicylate. Aspirin is the oldest NSAID, and has acted as the comparison for efficacy and adverse reactions. In recent years due to the association between Reye's syndrome and the use of salicylates during an antecedent illness, the use of aspirin and other salicylates is no longer recommended in the paediatric population except for juvenile rheumatoid disease where high doses of salicylates are used to relieve inflammation (75–90 mg/kg per day). These children are monitored closely for signs of salicylism, e.g. lethargy, emotional lability, tinnitus, or hyperpnoea. Aspartate aminotransferase and alanine aminotransferase should be monitored as with increasing serum levels the risk of hepatotoxicity increases. Salicylates are taken with food to minimize the risk of gastric irritation.

CONTRAINDICATIONS TO THE USE OF NSAIDS

The well-recognised contraindications to these drugs must be carefully observed in children (**Box 7.2**) and this gives particular problems in paediatrics where the incidence of asthma is rising. It is probably unwise to use these drugs in infants as renal maturation is still occurring in the first year of life. Paracetamol has been shown to be safe in infants and in those with renal compromise when used in an appropriate dose.

Contraindications to the use of NSAIDs in children

- infants less than one year of age
- children with regularly treated asthma or children in whom attacks of asthma, urticaria or acute rhinitis are precipitated by aspirin or other NSAIDs
- children with severe atopy
- nasal polyps
- dehydration or hypovolaemia for any reason
- renal impairment
- impaired hepatic function
- bleeding or coagulation disorders
- bleeding or peptic ulcer disease
- previous sensitivity to NSAIDs
- concurrent use of
  - other NSAIDs
  - other nephrotoxic agents, e.g. aminoglycosides
  - anticoagulants
- intraoperatively where there is a high risk of hemorrhage or large volume blood loss

Box 7.2

ADVERSE EFFECTS

While a study in the US in 1988 showed that approximately 6% of all drug reactions were associated with NSAID usage, only 1 in 6 of these occurred in people younger than 19 years of age. There is a low incidence of serious side effects overall, and while the number of adverse reactions has increased with increased usage in children the reports of serious consequences are rare. While some evidence suggests that some side effects are dose related, i.e. gastrointestinal, hepatic and renal side effects this does not appear to be the case in all patients. The most commonly reported side effects are gastrointestinal followed by skin, central nervous system, pulmonary, hepatic and renal toxic effects. Other serious side effects have been reported including oedema, bone marrow suppression, and Stevens–Johnson syndrome.

Gastrointestinal

The most commonly reported side effects following the use of NSAIDs are gastric irritation, gastritis and ulcerations, clinically presenting as upper dyspepsia, nausea and vomiting or even frank gastrointestinal bleeding. The reasons for this are many: local mucosal irritation, decreased mucus production and mucosal blood flow as well as increased gastric acid secretion resulting from a reduction in the local prostaglandin levels. There are NSAID preparations which incorporate prostaglandin analogues which minimize this effect. Avoiding the oral route may reduce these problems but does not eliminate them. H_2-blockers such as ranitidine may prevent some of these symptoms. Short term therapy with NSAIDs is less likely to induce symptoms. Occasionally transient abnormal liver function tests (elevated transaminases) have been reported in children.

Prolongation of bleeding time

In minor surgery the mild prolongation of bleeding time is not clinically significant. In major surgery, however, the NSAIDs should be used with caution and only commenced when primary clotting has already occurred.

Provocation of bronchospasm

Provocation of bronchospasm by NSAIDs is thought to be due to a relative excess of leukotriene production (the prostaglandin pathway is inhibited but the leuko-triene pathway is not leading to an imbalance). Though mainly seen with aspirin, cross-sensitivity with other NSAIDs is a definite possibility, especially as part of the syndrome of asthma, hay fever and nasal polyps. Those with multiple or severe allergies may also be at risk. Hence, in these children with definite asthma who are on regular preventative medication or who have been hospitalized with a severe attack (especially if this involved admission to intensive care) the NSAIDs are contraindicated. Caution is required in those with a less definite history, in those with severe eczema or multiple allergies and in those with nasal polyps.

Dermatological side effects

Dermatological side effects are often mild and variable. They are non-specific in nature including pruritis, hives, rash, erythema multiforme and phototoxic reactions. The mechanisms of these reactions are not well

179

understood. Children who developed photodermatitis were generally fair-skinned children who were receiving naproxen as treatment for juvenile rheumatoid arthritis. Active metabolites capable of initiating phototoxic reactions have also been shown with indomethacin and piroxicam. Phototoxic lesions are often subtle in nature and present as shallow ulcers. Treatment is by discontinuation of the drug.

Renal impairment

All the NSAIDs may lead to sodium, potassium and water retention, proteinuria and haematuria. Interstitial nephritis and acute renal failure have also been reported. Though mainly seen during long term NSAID therapy, these side effects have been reported in previously healthy and young adults. Pre-existing renal impairment may also increase the risk. The incidence of renal toxicity, however, appears to be low in children. The NSAIDs may result in a reduction of the local prostaglandin production in the kidneys. Under normal circumstances this is of less importance, but renal blood flow may depend on the production of local prostaglandins during anaesthesia or in cases where the circulating blood volume is reduced. Adequate hydration is important.

Documented renal papillary necrosis, demonstrated by intravenous pyelography, has also been diagnosed in a number of children being treated with non-steroidal anti-inflammatory drugs. These were children on long term treatment for juvenile rheumatoid arthritis who were treated with a variety of non-steroidals including indomethacin, naproxen and tolmetin. Therefore nephrotoxicity is a concern in the paediatric population especially in those with long term exposure. Other identifiable risk factors in the paediatric population are hypovolaemia secondary to salt depletion or restriction, or pre-existing renal disease. As the kidneys are still devloping in the first year of life, caution is required with NSAIDs in infants and many centres do not use this group of drugs in children aged < 1 year.

Other side effects

Effects on the bone marrow have been reported but are rare. They include aplastic anaemia, agranulocytosis, leukopenia and thrombocytopenia. Anaemia occurs in 2–14% of patients on prolonged therapy. Pulmonary oedema has occurred, mostly associated with aspirin. It is thought to be due to a diminished prostaglandin effect on the pulmonary microvasculature.

Headache, dizziness, tinnitus, decreased hearing, blurred vision and personality changes have been reported on rare occasions, especially following long term therapy with aspirin and indomethacin. NSAIDs can interact with other drugs (**Box 7.3**).

DRUG INTERACTIONS

Effect of NSAID interacting with other drugs	
Drug	Effect
Digoxin	Plasma concentration increased
Aminoglycosides	Plasma concentration increased
Valproate sodium	Plasma concentration increased (aspirin only)
Antihypertensives	Effect blunted by NSAIDs
Barbiturates	NSAIDs clearance is increased
Anticoagulants	Increased risk of GI bleeding

Box 7.3

PARACETAMOL
(ACETAMINOPHEN)

Paracetamol is the most popular analgesic in infants and children and has also been found to be safe and effective in neonates. The immaturity of hepatic metabolic systems in the newborn may be protective and leads to diminished production of the toxic metabolites of this drug. Its analgesic efficacy is equal to that of aspirin. It inhibits prostaglandin synthesis in the hypothalamus and so has an antipyretic effect, but does not have significant anti-inflammatory effects in the tissues. Doses of 15–20 mg/kg every 4–6 hours given orally produces therapeutic plasma concentrations of 10–25 mg/l, which is about 1/10th of the toxic plasma concentration threshold. The absorption from the rectal route is slow and it is now realized that higher loading doses of up to 45 mg/kg are required to achieve therapeutic plasma concentrations with subsequent rectal doses of 15–20 mg/kg 6–8 hourly for maintenance. Total daily doses of around 90 mg/kg/day can be used for up to 72 hours in otherwise healthy children as they are relatively resistant to hepatotoxicity. In neonates and young infants, 60 mg/kg/day is more appropriate with longer intervals between doses whether given rectally or orally.

Intravenous pro-paracetamol has been investigated in children and is commonly used in some European centres. Pro-paracetamol is rapidly hydrolysed in the body to paracetamol and the dose is twice that of the oral daily total given as a slow infusion over 15 minutes in four divided doses every 6 hours. Injection pain and hypotension are adverse effects seen with rapid bolus injection. (See **Box 7.4.**)

As paracetamol acts at a different site from the

Paracetamol dosage guidelines

Orally
   20 mg/kg loading dose, then 15 mg/kg 4–6 hourly to a maximum
   of 90 mg/kg/day (60 mg/kg/day in neonates)

Rectally
   30–45 mg/kg loading dose (20 mg/kg in neonates), then 20 mg/kg
   6–8 hourly to a maximum of 90 mg/kg/day (60 mg/kg/day in
   neonates)

Box 7.4

NSAIDs, the combination of paracetamol with NSAIDs produces an additive effect in terms of analgesia.

Paracetamol can cause severe hepatic necrosis in overdose. Paracetamol is extensively metabolized in the liver, the major metabolites being the sulphate and glucuronide conjugates. A minor fraction of the drug formed by P-450 metabolism is converted to a highly reactive alkylating metabolite which is then inactivated via glutathione conjugation and excreted in the urine as cysteine and mercapturic conjugates. Overdoses of paracetamol cause acute hepatic necrosis as a result of depletion of glutathione and of binding of the excess reactive metabolite to vital cell constituents.

NITROUS OXIDE
(see Chapter 9)

KEY LEARNING POINTS

● NSAIDs and paracetamol are useful for managing mild or moderate pain when given in appropriate doses

- in combination with local anaesthesia and/or opioids, they act synergistically to prevent and control moderate to severe pain
- the opioid sparing effect of NSAIDs and paracetamol is about 30% and concurrent administration allows more rapid weaning from opioids
- contraindications to NSAIDs and paracetamol should be carefully observed

FURTHER READING

Royal College of Paediatrics and Child Health (1997) *Prevention and Control of Pain in Children.* BMJ Publishing Group, London.

Montgomery C.J., McCormack J.P., Reichert C.C. and Marshland C.P. (1995) Plasma concentrations after high dose (45 mg/kg-1) rectal acetaminophen in children. *Canadian Journal of Anaesthesia* **42**, 982–986.

Henderson J.M., Spence D.G., Komocar L.M., Bonn G.E. and Stenstrom R.J. (1990) Administration of nitrous oxide to paediatric patients provides analgesia for venous cannulation. *Anaesthesiology* **72**, 269–271.

Joshi P., Ooi R. and Soni N. (1992) Nitrous oxide administration using commonly available oxygen therapy devices. *British Journal of Anaesthesia* **68**, 630–632.

CHAPTER 8

NON-PHARMACOLOGICAL TECHNIQUES

Kay O'Brien, Neil S. Morton

Principles

Cognitive and behavioural techniques

Transcutaneous electrical nerve stimulation (TENS)

PRINCIPLES

Most non-pharmacological techniques will not reduce the intensity of the pain but will help the child and parents to cope better and give a sense of being more in control. They should not usually be used instead of drug therapy but along with appropriate drugs.

COGNITIVE AND BEHAVIOURAL TECHNIQUES

Previously, management of paediatric pain was guided by the belief that a child's pain was directly proportional to the nature and extent of tissue damage. It is now realized that a child's age, sex, developmental level, prior pain experience and relevant psychological factors will affect how his or her nociceptive system responds to tissue damage. Situational factors vary extensively not only for different children experiencing the same tissue damage, but also for the same child experiencing the same tissue damage at different times. Therefore optimal pain control for children should include adequate analgesia administered at regular dosing intervals which ideally should be complemented by a consistent cognitive–behavioural approach.

Pain perception and response varies with age. There was a misconception that neonates do not feel pain and that they do not have a memory for pain which requires both the perception for pain and the cognitive capacity for memory. While it is difficult to show memory for pain there is ample evidence of cardiorespiratory, hormonal and behavioural responses that indicate pain. Expression of pain does alter with age with younger children responding by withdrawal and crying while older children are more likely to verbalize their distress. Children's cognitive development influences their pain in three ways. Firstly young children have a different understanding of the nature, treatment and cause of pain. Secondly, some treatments require levels of cognitive ability not available to younger children and thirdly, the way that children communicate about pain as above depends on their cognitive development. Irrespective of developmental level, children remain relatively poorly informed about the nature of pain, its significance for them, and what they can do to cope with it. Behavioural factors also have a powerful role in children's pain with some behaviours promoting a healthy recovery, while others initiate, exacerbate or maintain children's pain. When children lack understanding, control and positive coping behaviours, their emotional distress increases and their pain intensifies.

COMMON FACTORS THAT INCREASE CHILDREN'S PAIN
PERCEPTION. See Box 8.1

Cognitive interventions are probably the most important and versatile non-pharmacological pain therapies for children.

INFORMATION

Accurate age-appropriate information about a pain source or procedure provides a practical, effective method for relieving a child's distress.

DISTRACTION

The distraction technique is an active process that can reduce the neuronal responses to a noxious stimulus. Children are not simply ignoring their pain, but are reducing their perception of it. Parents and staff can play an important part in distraction techniques by

Common factors that exacerbate children's pain	
Situational	Insufficient information
	Lack of perceived patient control
	Few non-pharmacological means of pain control available to patient
	Previously learned pain triggers
Behavioural	Obvious distress of carers/parents
	Inconsistent parental responses
	Prolonged physical distress (secondary gain)
	Limited physical activity
	Limited social activity
Emotional	Specific fears of diagnosis/treatment
	General anxiety

Box 8.1

helping the child to concentrate fully on objects, events or sounds as opposed to concentrating on their pain. Play therapists can have a major input by encouraging social interaction and teaching play skills to younger children. Comfort blankets or toys, jokes, games, puzzles, blowing bubbles, kaleidoscopes, headphones with stories or music, or reading books (especially interactive ones) can all be used. The introduction of interactive computer and video games has also provided a tool that can be used successfully by parents and staff. Stimulation of the major senses is the key, after an assessment of what the child finds interesting.

PHYSIOTHERAPY
Physical therapy reduces pain by stimulating different body regions and selectively stimulating non-nociceptive afferents. Most people have rubbed a painful area to decrease pain with good effect. Even simple stretching a few times a week maintains flexibility and allows children to actively participate in their own pain management programmes, allowing them more control over their treatment and decreasing their dependence on medications and on parents.

RELAXATION
Acute pain during invasive treatments may be decreased by simple exercise and relaxation therapy. Simple techniques like deep breathing, rhythmically moving a leg or loosening a fist can relax other body parts and dramatically reduce procedural pain. This type of behavioural therapy is aimed at the children themselves again increasing their control over the situation.

IMAGERY

An extension of this is to guide the child through an imaginary journey or favourite activity, e.g. football, horse riding, basketball. The key moment such as scoring a goal can coincide with the painful procedure for maximum benefit. Hypnosis is another similar technique of focussing attention to distract the child from perceiving pain.

MASSAGE AND TOUCH

Massage and touch are commonly used to aid relaxation and to comfort children. This is particularly useful in distressed children and small babies.

SUMMARY

In summary, children's pain is influenced by many factors, no matter how obvious the aetiology. Therefore pain control must be addressed from a multidimensional perspective. Regular analgesia must be administered at regular dosing intervals, and treatment should also provide a practical cognitive–behavioural approach (**Box 8.2**). Situational, behavioural and emotional factors must all be addressed to ensure optimum treatment for the child.

TRANSCUTANEOUS ELECTRICAL NERVE STIMULATION (TENS)

Transcutaneous electrical nerve stimulation (TENS) is widely used in the treatment of adult chronic pain with good effect. More recently it has been shown to reduce analgesic requirements and subjective reports of pain after some operations. It is often useful in the treatment

---

Objectives of cognitive–behavioural programme

1. Provision of accurate information to child and parents with regard to pain problems and the factors that modify pain perception
2. Removal of situational factors that increase pain
   - reduce waiting time for theatre or ward procedures if possible
   - increase physical activity
   - increase patient involvement in pain management, decreasing reliance on parents and medications
   - reduce anxiety-related pain behaviour
3. Teach patients active methods of reducing or coping with pain
4. Provide a consistent approach from medical staff and parents encouraging children to be actively involved in their pain management

Box 8.2

of neuropathic pain which is poorly responsive to opioids. TENS is normally used in combination with other modes of pain relief and not as a sole agent. TENS has been shown to decrease procedural pain in children, the effect being greatest in older children. Children and adults with a psychological or social component to their pain had a poorer response to treatment using TENS.

It is difficult to fully understand the neurophysiological basis of TENS. Pain is mediated through the unmyelinated C fibres and the lightly myelinated A-alpha fibres. Large diameter fibres transmit impulses at a faster speed than those of the unmyelinated or lighter myelinated fibres.

Low frequency, high intensity TENS of less than 10 Hz has been clinically shown to create analgesia. Endorphins have been created in the absence of pain, and the effect of TENS has been eliminated by simultaneous use of nalaxone, an indication of a neurochemical basis. Electrical stimulation has also been shown to decrease the nerve action potential of A-delta fibres, which are pain mediators. All these factors confirm a physiological basis for effective pain modulation. However, the manner, site and type of TENS is vital for effective pain modulation. There are two common modes of TENS: (1) conventional, which is the type frequently used in post-operative pain management and (2) acupuncture-like.

CONVENTIONAL TENS

Conventional TENS uses high frequency currents, i.e. $\cong$ 100 Hz, which stimulates the large myelinated A-beta fibres. This closes the 'gates' in the dorsal horn and inhibits transmission of pain impulses along the small diameter, pain transmitting C and A-delta fibres. Conventional TENS is effective immediately on starting treatment. Some TENS machines have a 'bolus' or 'boost' facility with a button similar to a PCA pump. Acupuncture-like TENS uses the lower frequency currents, i.e. < 10 Hz, which are thought to stimulate the production and release of endorphins. As this process takes some time, the onset of pain relief with this method may take up to 60 minutes. The use of TENS is simple, non-invasive and user friendly, giving the patient some control over their treatment. The technique is quickly learnt by older children and is virtually free from side effects. The patient is provided with a small battery-powered TENS unit which generates a small electric current that is transmitted via electrodes placed on the skin. Maximum effect is achieved by placing the electrodes over the nerve innervating the affected area, over the affected dermatome or as close as is possible, above and below the painful area or over trigger or acupuncture sites. The patient may then vary the amplitude and frequency of the current delivered according to the severity of the pain and its response. The current should be altered to produce an easily tolerated tingling sensation or buzzing on the skin. TENS should be avoided in patients with cardiac pacemakers as it may cause electrical interference. Mild skin irritation may occur so the electrode sites should be regularly inspected.

FEEDING: 'MILK' OR 'SUCROSE' ANALGESIA

Feeding a small baby often induces a deep settled sleep pattern which may allow mildly painful procedures to be performed, such as removal of a dressing or superficial sutures. The feed probably stimulates production of the child's own endogenous opioids which have analgesic and sedative properties. A similar effect is seen in small infants when a sweet sucrose solution is placed on the tongue and the distress caused by needling procedures is reduced, e.g. capillary heel sampling, venepuncture or spinal or caudal anaesthesia in the awake baby.

KEY LEARNING POINTS

- the definition of pain demonstrates that there are emotional and physical components which must be addressed in treating pain effectively
- assessment of children must include a judgement about which non-drug methods will be practicable and helpful
- early institution of physiotherapy, play therapy and psychology input to management of children's pain is very beneficial and often reduces drug requirements.

FURTHER READING

Brereton K. (1997) Non-pharmacological pain management. *Manual of Acute Pain Management in Children.* pp. 101–108. Churchill Livingstone, London.

Lander J. and Fowler-Kerry S. (1993) TENS for children's procedural pain. *Pain* **52**, 209–216.

Twycross A. (1998) Paediatric pain management – a multi disciplinary approach. Radcliffe Medical Press, Oxford.

CHAPTER 9

SAFE SEDATION OF CHILDREN FOR THERAPEUTIC AND DIAGNOSTIC PROCEDURES

Neil S. Morton

Aims and problems

Definitions

Principles of safe sedation of children

Patient selection

Patient preparation

Monitoring standards

Recommended techniques

Sedation plans for specific procedures

The actual figures of mortality and morbidity in children under sedation are not known. In an analysis of sedation disasters in the United States, 52 deaths and 27 cases of significant morbidity were reported which were directly attributed to sedation. These were mainly due to drug overdose, inadequate monitoring, inadequate training or premature discharge home. In a recent survey of paediatric sedation practice in Scotland only 3 out of 38 hospital departments who sedate children had a formal protocol for paediatric sedation while 7 of the 163 respondents said they always used general anaesthesia for diagnostic or therapeutic procedures in children. One third did not fast children at all prior to sedation

and one third did not secure venous access when sedating children; 1 in 5 did not have comprehensive resuscitation equipment and in 1 in 6 locations, no monitoring
was used. Only 1 in 5 units assessed sedation level.
Midazolam was the most common sedative agent used
and local anaesthesia was used by two thirds of the
respondents. One third of the departments who under-
took paediatric sedation had encountered problems
owing to inadequate sedation or oversedation, and 1 in
9 reported morbidity with paediatric sedation. Very few
units document the sedation procedure and vital signs
adequately and this may have medicolegal implications
especially if something goes wrong during the procedure
or if the child is inadequately sedated and suffers distress
from the procedure. It is important to realize that
hospitals and practitioners are being taken to task in
court for inadequate sedation as well as for 'sedation
disasters'.

AIMS AND PROBLEMS

The aims of sedating children for diagnostic or therapeutic procedures are to relieve anxiety and stress, to
provide pain relief, to induce appropriate sleep and to
keep the child still enough to allow safe conduct of the
procedure. The problems in achieving these aims are
primarily the wide variability in response of children to
sedative agents in terms of both dose requirements and
clinical effects. There is a continuum from the awake to
the anaesthetized state with loss of protective airway
reflexes occurring unpredictably. Hypoventilation,
apnoea and airway obstruction may occur with hypoxaemia and hypercarbia developing. This is particularly

seen in younger infants or where combinations of sedatives and opioids are used. Cardiac output, heart rate
and blood pressure may fall with development of metabolic acidosis. Pulmonary, intracranial and intraocular
pressures may rise primarily owing to the effects of the
sedative drug, e.g. ketamine, or secondarily to hypoxaemia, acidosis and hypercarbia. Disinhibition, restlessness and movement can occur unpredictably and may be
exacerbated by hypoxaemia. Progression of the depth of
sedation after painful or stimulating procedures are
finished is also commonly seen particularly when long
acting agents are used. To achieve the aims of sedation
while minimizing the problems is difficult and in some
children should not be attempted (see patient selection
below).

DEFINITIONS

Sedation is defined as a technique in which the use of a
drug or drugs produces a state of depression of the
central nervous system enabling treatment to be carried
out, *but during which verbal contact with the patient is
maintained* throughout the period of sedation. The
drugs and techniques used should carry a margin of
safety wide enough to render unintended loss of consciousness unlikely. In the sedated state, protective
reflexes are maintained, the airway is maintained independently and continuously and the child can respond
to physical stimulation or verbal command.

In children it is difficult to achieve adequate anxiolysis, analgesia, sleep and lack of movement to allow the
safe conduct of many diagnostic and therapeutic procedures if a state of sedation as defined in this way is used.

Many children are in fact *anaesthetized* to achieve these aims. Loss of consciousness is a state of anaesthesia with all its attendant risks. In the anaesthetized child, partial or complete loss of protective reflexes occurs, the airway cannot be maintaned independently and continuously and the child is unable to to respond to physical stimulation or verbal command. To try to differentiate light sedation, deep sedation and anaesthesia is fundamentally flawed because the states overlap unpredictably.

PRINCIPLES OF SAFE SEDATION OF CHILDREN

The standards of care of the sedated child should therefore be those of the child undergoing general anaesthesia. This requires careful selection and preparation of patients, exclusion of unsuitable patients, use of appropriate drugs, equipment, clinical and electronic monitoring by personnel appropriately trained in paediatric sedation and resuscitation, avoidance of the 'operator-sedationist' and implementation of appropriate discharge criteria. This is the approach recommended in adult practice by the working party reports of several Royal Colleges (of Physicians, Surgeons, Anaesthetists, Radiologists and Ophthalmologists) and in the published guidelines from the American Academy of Paediatrics. A rational approach is to ask and answer certain key questions (**Box 9.1**) before undertaking the procedure.

It is preferable to use drugs with a rapid onset and short duration of action so that titration of the dose to achieve the desired effect is easier. The ability to pharmacologically antagonize any sedatives used is desirable.

▼ **Rational approach to paediatric sedation**

- is the procedure going to be painful?
- how long will the procedure last?
- what is the medical status and age of the child?
- are there contraindications to sedation?
- has consent been obtained?
- has the child been fasted?
- who is going to look after the child during and after the period of sedation?
- what training does this person have?
- when and by whom is the child going to be discharged?

Box 9.1

If the procedure is painful use of local anaesthesia at the painful site applied topically in advance and/or infiltrated has an important 'sedative-sparing' effect and often circumvents the need for opioids with all their potential adverse effects.

PATIENT SELECTION

A full history and examination should be carried out and an active search made for contraindications to sedation and for significant underlying medical and surgical disorders (**Box 9.2**). The past sedation history should be checked because previous failed sedation may warrant referral for a general anaesthetic. Small children merit particular caution and in some children the pharmacokinetics and dynamics of sedatives may be abnormal, e.g. in renal failure and in hepatic failure and in children with induced enzymes such as those on regular anticonvulsant drugs (**Box 9.3**).

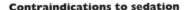
Contraindications to sedation

- abnormal airway
- raised intracranial pressure
- depressed conscious level
- history of sleep apnoea
- respiratory failure
- cardiac failure
- gastro-oesophageal reflux
- bowel obstruction
- active infection
- known drug allergy/adverse reaction
- previous failed sedation

Box 9.2

Particular caution required with sedation

- neonate, especially if premature or ex-premature
- infants and children age < 5 years
- renal impairment
- hepatic impairment
- epilepsy
- on anticonvulsant therapy
- asthma

Box 9.3

PATIENT PREPARATION

Written informed consent should be obtained and this should include an explanation of the procedure and sedation technique to be used. Parents should be informed of the possibility that sedation may fail and that either the procedure may have to be abandoned or the child may require a formal general anaesthetic. The child should be fasted as for a general anaesthetic (6 hours for solids or bottle milk, 4 hours for breast milk, 3 hours for clear fluids). Venous access should be secured under topical local anaesthetic cover if at all possible prior to the administration of any sedation. Topical local anaesthesia should also be applied to the sites of any other needle punctures such as for lumbar puncture, bone marrow sampling or cannulation for interventional radiology or cardiology. The skin overlying these areas will be anaesthetized and the area can then be infiltrated with further local anaesthetic prior to the needling procedure. The sedative prescription should be double-checked to ensure dosages are correct. Monitoring should be started from the time of administration of the sedative agent until discharge and this must include the period when the patient is being transferred, e.g. from ward to radiology department. Equipment for monitoring children and paediatric resuscitation drugs and equipment must be available throughout the period from the time the sedative is given until discharge. The staff undertaking this monitoring role must be properly trained and should be able to deliver basic life support measures and initiate advanced life support for children. (See **Box 9.4**.)

MONITORING STANDARDS

The personnel undertaking monitoring of the sedated child must be appropriately trained in paediatric resuscitation, monitoring techniques and sedation techniques. These individuals may be nursing, paediatric medical, surgical, radiology or anaesthetic staff and should have

Checklist for safe paediatric sedation

- check age, weight and identity
- check consent
- check fasting
- check for contraindications
- check past sedation history
- check for significant underlying medical or surgical disorders
- check for allergies
- double-check the sedation prescription and administration
- check monitoring, resuscitation equipment and drugs
- check the supervision of the child from pre-sedation to discharge

Box 9.4

as their *sole* duty the monitoring of the sedated child and should not take part in the procedure. They must be *additional* to and separate from the person carrying out the procedure whether this is diagnostic or therapeutic. In some countries the concept of monitored anaesthesia care has been developed for such situations and it may be that anaesthetists need to become more actively involved in the large numbers of such cases. The most important monitor is the trained person using observational and clinical skills and assisted by electronic monitoring as appropriate (e.g. pulse oximetry, ECG, non-invasive blood pressure device, temperature measurement and capnography).

The frequency and intensity of observations and assessments to be made should be matched to the child and the procedure and a balance must be struck between safety and practicality to allow the procedure to proceed without arousing the sleeping child and with the minimum of disruption. A suggested scheme is given in **Figure 9.1** and it is important for clinical and legal reasons that the observations are charted, something that is rarely done in many centres at present. The minimum monitoring standard should comprise regular assessments of the level of sedation, oxygen saturation by pulse oximetry, respiratory rate and pulse rate supplemented by temperature, ECG and blood pressure for infants, for prolonged procedures or where verbal contact with the child is lost. Monitoring should continue after the procedure, during transfer back to the recovery or ward area until discharge criteria are met (**Box 9.5**). This is important because the depth of sedation may progress particularly after the stimulus of a painful procedure has receded and especially if long acting agents are used. A proactive check on the patency and stability of the airway should be made, protective reflexes should be intact, the child should be awake or back to his normal response level, hydration should be adequate and haemodynamics should be stable.

Recovery and discharge criteria

- airway patent and stable unsupported
- easily rousable
- oxygen saturation >96% breathing air
- haemodynamically stable
- hydration adequate
- returned to normal level of responsiveness and orientation for age and mental status
- can talk (age appropriate)
- can sit up unaided (age appropriate)

Box 9.5

ROYAL HOSPITAL FOR SICK CHILDREN, GLASGOW
SEDATION MONITORING: MEDICAL CHECK LIST

NAME: DOB: AGE: years   months
HOSPITAL NO:
RESPONSIBLE CONSULTANT: WARD:
PROCEDURE:
Elective / Urgent / Emergency *(Please circle)*
DIAGNOSIS: WEIGHT: kg

Check for Contraindications to Sedation (if YES seek advice from Consultant)

Airway compromised	YES	NO
Raised intracranial pressure	YES	NO
Depressed conscious level	YES	NO
History of sleep apnoea	YES	NO
Respiratory failure	YES	NO

Past Sedation History:

Previous sedation   YES NO
Satisfactory   YES NO
Specify:
Previous failed sedation YES NO Reason:
Previous complications of sedation, specify:

Check Fasting Time

Fasted for solids (including milk) from: (insert time) (minimum 6 hours)
Fasted for breast milk from: (insert time) (minimum 4 hours)

204

Fasted for juice/water from: (insert time) (minimum 3 hours)

Check for Significant Underlying Surgical or Medical Disorders (if YES seek advice from Consultant)

Renal dysfunction	YES	NO
Liver dysfunction	YES	NO
Respiratory dysfunction	YES	NO
Cardiac dysfunction	YES	NO
Active infection	YES	NO
(esp. upper/lower respiratory tract infection)		
History of gastro-oesophageal reflux	YES	NO
Known allergies/Drug reactions	YES	NO

Sedation prescription:

DRUG: DOSE: TIME:

Check Supervision of Sedated Child:

Name Position

Who is the qualified attendant:

Who is accompanying child in transit:

Check Equipment

Pulse Oximeter ECG BP Temp Oxygen Suction Airway Equip Circulatory Support

Equipment Resusc Drugs Venous Access Defib

Signature of Doctor Block Capitals Position Date

Figure 9.1
Checklist and monitoring chart for paediatric sedation

ROYAL HOSPITAL FOR SICK CHILDREN •
SEDATION MONITORING CHART

PRIOR TO PROCEDURE : RECORD sedation score with an X, SpO$_2$, RR, HR

DURING PROCEDURE : RECORD sedation score as Ⓐ every 15 minutes if
formally assessed level of sedation

: RECORD SpO$_2$, RR, HR every 5 minutes (add Temp
score 2 or more)

: RECORD Sedation score with an X after formally as
means interrupting investigation)

AFTER PROCEDURE: : CONTINUE TO RECORD sedation score (X), SpO
indicated) until sedation score 1 or 0 for three succe

INSERT TIME		:00 05 10	15 20 25	30 35 40	45 50 55	:00 05 10	15 20 25	30 35 40
SEDATION SCORE								
Eyes open spont = 0								
Eyes open to speech = 1								
Eyes open to shake = 2								
Unrousable = 3								
SpO$_2$ %								
RR bpm								
HR bpm								
BP	DIA							
	SYS							
Temp °C								

Signature of trained observers:
PRIOR TO PROCEDURE .... Sig .... Block cap .... Date

DURING TRANSIT .... Sig .... Block cap .... Date

206

GLASGOW

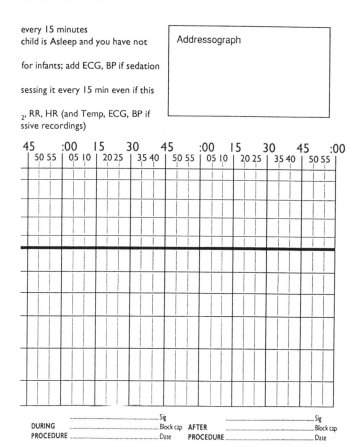

every 15 minutes
child is Asleep and you have not

for infants; add ECG, BP if sedation

sessing it every 15 min even if this

$_2$, RR, HR (and Temp, ECG, BP if
ssive recordings)

Addressograph

Figure 9.1 (continued)

RECOMMENDED TECHNIQUES

Single short acting sedative agents (e g midazolam) and appropriate use of local anaesthesia (topically applied and/or infiltrated) are preferred. Combinations of sedatives with opioids and use of long acting agents are not recommended. Anaesthetic drugs such as propofol or ketamine should only be given by anaesthetists.

NITROUS OXIDE OR ENTONOX

Nitrous oxide is a gas with analgesic and sedative properties which is taken up and eliminated very rapidly from the lungs. It is very insoluble in the blood so is delivered very quickly to the brain to produce an analgesic effect equivalent to intravenous morphine. Maximal pain relief is achieved after approximately 2 minutes of inhalation. Nitrous oxide can be given in oxygen in inspired concentrations up to 70% but this requires a special delivery system and this concentration may lead to loss of verbal contact with the patient. It is more conveniently given in the form of 'Entonox' which is a cylinder of premixed nitrous oxide in oxygen which automatically delivers 50% nitrous oxide and 50% oxygen. The cylinder contents are under pressure and a flow of gas to the patient is usually activated on demand by the patient taking a breath in via a special valve. Recently the design of these valves has improved to a lightweight, child-friendly system with an opening pressure of 1–2 cm of water. The child can breath via a facemask, nasal mask or mouthpiece and the system is best regarded as a form of inhaled PCA with the child holding the mask or mouthpiece and controlling the inhalation. This has an important safety function in maintaining sedation and thus verbal contact. It is not very suitable for children less than 3 years old and works best of all in cooperative children aged more than 5 years. Entonox can be used for a wide variety of procedures in paediatrics which require potent analgesia for a short time (**Box 9.6**).

Nitrous oxide is not suitable for all children and there are absolute contraindications to its administration (**Box 9.7**).

Uses for nitrous oxide/Entonox

- suture insertion or removal
- dressing removal or changes (including burns)
- drain or catheter removal
- venepuncture or cannulation
- lumbar puncture
- physiotherapy
- biopsies (skin, muscle, renal, bone marrow)

Box 9.6

Absolute contraindications to nitrous oxide/Entonox

- pneumothorax
- bowel obstruction
- abnormal airway
- recent head injury (especially if intracranial air)
- chronic respiratory disease
- uncorrected congenital heart disease
- gastro-oesophageal reflux
- age < 3 years
- cannot cooperate or understand technique
- previous problems with Entonox

Box 9.7

ROYAL HOSPITAL FOR SICK CHILDREN • GLASGOW
ENTONOX ANALGESIA: MEDICAL CHECK LIST

Name: DOB: WEIGHT: kg

Hospital Number: AGE: years   months

Ward:

Responsible Consultant:

Diagnosis:

Procedure requiring Entonox Analgesia:

Check for Contraindications to Entonox

Age: < 1 year	YES	NO
Airway abnormality	YES	NO
Breathing : history of sleep apnoea	YES	NO
: respiratory disease	YES	NO
: active upper / lower respiratory infection	YES	NO
Conscious level: depressed	YES	NO
Raised intracranial pressure	YES	NO
Recent head injury	YES	NO
Pneumothorax	YES	NO
Bowel obstruction	YES	NO
History of gastro-oesophageal reflux	YES	NO
Uncorrected congenital heart disease	YES	NO

Check Fasting Time

Fasting for solids / bottle milk	from:	(Insert time) (minimum 6 hours)
Fasting for breast milk	from:	(Insert time) (minimum 4 hours)
Fasting for clear fluids	from:	(Insert time) (minimum 3 hours)

Past Entonox history: (specify)

Other sedatives being given at present: (specify)

Check supervision of child:

	Name	Position

Who is the trained Entonox administrator:

Who is carrying out procedure:

This is a single Entonox administration / This is part of a series of Entonox administrations

Check Equipment:

Pulse Oximeter: Entonox apparatus:

Oxygen apparatus:

Suction apparatus:

Resuscitation equipment:

Resuscitation drugs:

.... Signature of Doctor
.... Block Capitals
.... Position
.... Date
.... Time

Figure 9.2
Entonox selection checklist and monitoring chart

211

ROYAL HOSPITAL FOR SICK CHILDREN •
ENTONOX MONITORING CHART

INSERT TIME	:00	05	10	15	20	25	30	35	40	45	50	55	:00	05	10	15	20	25	30	35	40
SpO$_2$ %																					
Sedation Score Eyes open spont = 0 Eyes open to speech = 1 Eyes open to shake = 2 Unrousable = 3																					
Pain Score 0-3																					
Nausea Score 0-3																					
Respiratory Rate																					

Signature of trained observer ....

Block capitals ....

Date ....

Time ....

GLASGOW

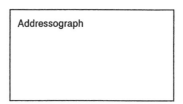

Addressograph

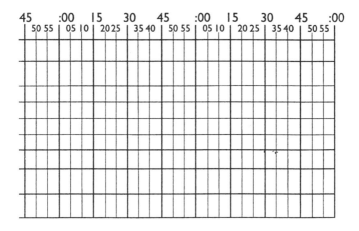

45		:00		15		30		45		:00		15		30		45		:00
	50 55		05 10		20 25		35 40		50 55		05 10		20 25		35 40		50 55	

Figure 9.2 (continued)

Nitrous oxide is highly diffusable and will move more rapidly into an air pocket than the nitrogen in the air pocket moves out. The air pocket will therefore expand in volume or if in a confined space (e.g. within the chest or cranial cavities or within the lumen of the bowel) the pressure will increase. This tension effect is extremely dangerous producing tension pneumothorax, ischaemia or shift of intracranial contents or bowel distension with risk of perforation.

Nitrous oxide produces a degree of sedation and potentiates the sedative effects of other central nervous system depressants, so care is required when opioids, benzodiazepines, antihistamines, etc., have also been given. Nitrous oxide can also induce nausea and vomiting but if it is to be used as the sole sedative and analgesic, the incidence of emesis is very low and therefore fasting is not required. If, however, other sedatives or analgesics have been given, the child should be fasted as for a general anaesthetic (6 hours for solids or milk, 3 hours for clear fluids). Other adverse effects of nitrous oxide are the potential to oxidize vitamin B12 and affect erythropoiesis and these are disputed effects on personnel of prolonged or repeated exposure. It is important that nitrous oxide administration is performed in well-ventilated areas and that where possible the expired gases are scavenged.

As with any sedative technique, consent, selection, preparation, monitoring and record keeping should be as noted above and trained personnel should be in charge of administering and monitoring the child receiving nitrous oxide. A simplified monitoring chart is shown in Figure 9.2.

MIDAZOLAM

Midazolam is a water-soluble benzodiazepine which produces sedation, anxiolysis and amnesia but is not an analgesic. It can be administered by parenteral (iv, im), oral, sublingual, nasal or rectal routes.

It is rapidly distributed and has an elimination half-life of 70–140 minutes but this is considerably prolonged in neonates.

Intravenous midazolam

The intravenous formulation of midazolam (2 or 5 mg/ml) is very acidic with a pH of 3.3 and prior to administration to children it is advisable to dilute the drug with 5% dextrose or 0.9% saline to a minimum volume of 10 ml. There is no pain on injection and small increments of 0.05 mg/kg (50 micrograms/kg) given over 10–15 seconds will produce smooth induction of sedation whilst minimizing respiratory depression or hypotension. The onset of action is slower than that seen with intravenous anaesthetic agents and this means that after each increment a delay of at least 60 seconds should be allowed for the effects of the drug to be seen. The incremental dose of 0.05 mg/kg can be repeated in this way, titrating the dose against the level of sleep up to a total dose of 0.3 mg/kg. A useful clinical end point for a safe level of sedation is ptosis (closure of the eyelids).

Occasionally, hypotension is seen when bolus doses are used in critically ill or very small infants and particular care is required in these cases. Respiratory depression may be seen, particularly when midazolam is given along with opioids or other sedative agents. Like all benzodiazepines, midazolam can produce a state of disinhibition or restlessness in up to 10% of children, especially in those less than 5 years of age. This state does not respond to further increments of the drug and misinterpretation of this sign can lead to overdosage of the drug.

There is a wide interpatient variability in response to benzodiazepines, so titration with an upper dose limit is the safest approach. The intravenous midazolam technique must only be used in the context of careful patient selection, preparation and monitoring and children must be fasted as if they are having a general anaesthetic. This procedure must not be undertaken by untrained staff. The person giving intravenous midazolam must be fully trained in paediatric sedation and paediatric resuscitation and must have as their sole duty the sedation and monitoring of the child. They must not undertake the diagnostic or therapeutic procedure as well. Trained anaesthetic or medical staff or nurse specialists can all use this technique safely provided the selection and monitoring standards are implemented correctly.

Oral midazolam

Midazolam can be given orally and this route has been extensively researched as a method of premedication of children. The standard intravenous formulation is used but is very bitter tasting, so a sweet vehicle is required as disguise. A variety of local favourite formulations have been developed including standard pharmaceutical syrup, cola, lemonade, sweet or iced fruit juices, paracetamol syrup or a Glasgow perennial, 'Irn-Bru'™! Up to 1 ml/kg of any of these can be allowed as a diluent and a commercially produced formulation is under trial. The oral dose is ten times larger than the intravenous incremental dose because of extensive first-pass liver metabolism after gastrointestinal absorption. The most commonly used dose is 0.5 mg/kg, maximum 15 mg (although some workers recommend 0.75 mg/kg). The onset of effect is within 30 minutes and there is a further 30 minute window of opportunity when sedation is at its maximum. Supplementary intravenous midazolam may be given, with the provisos noted above. For painful procedures, local anaesthesia supplementation should be used in preference to opioid supplementation to minimize the risk of respiratory depression. In some cases, nitrous oxide/Entonox analgesia may be more appropriate.

Recovery after these techniques is rapid and is usually complete within two hours, allowing early return to oral intake of fluids and nutrition and prompt discharge home if appropriate.

Midazolam-based sedation techniques should be the first choice technique in modern paediatric practice and a suggested scheme to cover most paediatric diagnostic and therapeutic procedures is outlined in **Figure 9.3**.

ANTAGONISM OF BENZODIAZEPINE SEDATION WITH FLUMAZENIL

In the event of overdosage with midazolam, basic and advanced life support measures are the priority (Airway, Breathing, Circulation, Oxygen) but the specific benzodiazepine antagonist flumazenil should also be considered. Flumazenil must be available immediately whenever midazolam is given to children. The incremental dose is 5 micrograms/kg, repeated every 60 seconds to a total of 40 micrograms/kg. In severe cases, an infusion of flumazenil may be needed as its effective half-life is shorter than most of the benzodiazepines (rate 10 micrograms/kg/hr). Children receiving flumazenil may awaken very abruptly and may become

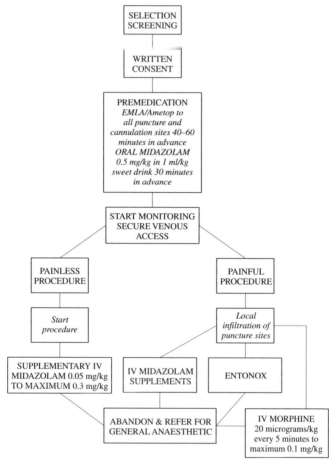

Figure 9.3
Suggested sedation regimen (note the use of reversible agents)

acutely agitated, restless or even have seizures, and care must be taken to protect the child from injury if this occurs. The availability of flumazenil should not be an excuse for using excessive doses of benzodiazepines and care is required when deciding when to discharge children if flumazenil has been used, as resedation is a possibility owing to the longer duration of action of most benzodiazepines when compared to that of flumazenil.

Midazolam can also be given by the nasal, rectal or intramuscular routes but these are unpleasant and disliked by children and cannot be recommended.

TEMAZEPAM

Temazepam can be used orally as anxiolytic and sedative premedication prior to procedures in a dose of 0.2–0.5 mg/kg to a maximum dose of 20 mg. It is best given 60–90 minutes in advance of the procedure and produces useful sedation for up to 2 hours. The syrup (1 mg/kg) or tablet formulations can be used.

DIAZEPAM

Diazepam can be useful as oral premedication in a dose of 0.2–0.3 mg/kg. As an emulsion formulation it can be titrated intravenously in increments of 0.1 mg/kg repeated at 60 second intervals up to a total maximum dose of 0.5 mg/kg or until ptosis is seen. Diazepam has a long acting active metabolite which may delay recovery. The effects of diazepam can be reversed by flumazenil as above.

TRIMEPRAZINE

Trimeprazine oral syrup is still commonly used as a paediatric sedative, antiemetic premedication. The recommended dose is 1–2 mg/kg, but many paediatric centres still use 3 mg/kg. Recovery may be prolonged after larger doses. Sedation is not reversible with flumazenil or naloxone.

219

CHLORAL HYDRATE

This syrup is used for sedative premedication prior to non-painful procedures. The recommended dose is 25–50 mg/kg but doses up to 100 mg/kg are sometimes used. The onset of sedation takes about 1 hour and lasts about 1 hour, but residual effects may be evident for 24 hours. Particular care is required when combined with other sedative agents. Gastric irritation, hypotension and excessive depth of sedation may occur and the sedation is not reversible with flumazenil or naloxone.

BARBITURATES

Rectally or orally administered barbiturates (e.g. oral quinalbarbitone 5–10 mg/kg) have been used for paediatric sedation but produce variable depth and duration of sedation. They should not be used for painful procedures. There are no antagonists available.

KETAMINE

Ketamine is an anaesthetic agent which can be given by the oral, intravenous or intramuscular routes. It should only be administered by trained anaesthetists and children should be fasted as for a general anaesthetic. In low doses it is a potent analgesic and in higher doses it also produces a state of dissociative anaesthesia. Ketamine tends to cause sympathetic nervous system stimulation and so blood pressure tends to remain stable or increases, intracranial pressure increases and elevated pulmonary pressure may rise further. It should not be used in patients with systemic, intracranial or pulmonary hypertension. Ketamine induces dose-related respiratory depression and augments the respiratory depressant effects of other sedative agents. It also tends to stimulate salivation and airway secretions and this may induce coughing and laryngeal spasm. These effects can be prevented by atropine premedication (orally 20–40 micrograms/kg or iv 10–20 micrograms/kg). Central nervous stimulation may lead to restlessness, nightmares and delirium but these effects can be reduced by premedication with a benzodiazepine as above. The new purified stereoisomer form of ketamine (*S*-ketamine) is as effective as ketamine without producing the CNS side effects (**Table 9.1**).

OPIOIDS

Opioids should only be used for painful procedures where local anaesthesia cannot be used or has failed. They should not be used as sedatives for non-painful procedures because of the risk of respiratory depression. Cocktails of sedatives with opioids given orally or intramuscularly should not be used as they are associated with a high risk of respiratory depression, loss of airway control, cardiovascular instability and prolonged recovery. Short acting potent opioids such as fentanyl, alfentanil and remifentanil should only be used by anaesthetists or intensivists and should not be used outwith the operating room or intensive care unit. It is probably best to become familiar with titrating one opioid such as morphine given in small increments intravenously, e.g. 20 micrograms/kg, repeated every 5

Table 9.1 Ketamine dosage schedule

Oral: 10–20 mg/kg, 20–30 minutes in advance
Intramuscular: 2–10 mg/kg
Intravenous: 1–2 mg/kg, increments 0.5 mg/kg every 60 seconds or infusion 10–50 micrograms/kg/min

minutes to the desired end point. Morphine can be given orally but the sedative effect can be unpredictable and it is difficult to titrate the dose to achieve the desired effect.

ANTAGONIST FOR OPIOIDS: NALOXONE

The sedative, respiratory depressant and analgesic effects of opioids can be antagonized by naloxone 2–4 micrograms/kg iv repeated to 10 micrograms/kg. The duration of naloxone's effect is short and an infusion may have to be given to maintain reversal at a dose of 10 micrograms/kg/hr. Naloxone can be given IM in an emergency in a dose of 10 micrograms/kg.

SEDATION PLANS FOR SPECIFIC PROCEDURES
(see Chapter 10)

KEY LEARNING POINTS

- children undergoing sedation should be prepared and monitored as for a general anaesthetic
- a separate trained person should monitor the child during and after sedation
- the contraindications to sedation must be actively sought
- an accurate record of the sedation procedure and monitored recordings should be made and filed in the case record
- single titratable antagonizable agents should be used and combinations with opioids avoided
- do not use opioids for non-painful procedures
- use local anaesthesia for pain control wherever possible

FURTHER READING

Royal College of Paediatrics and Child Health (1997) *Prevention and Control of Pain in Children.* BMJ Publishing Group, London.

Committee on Drugs (1992) Guidelines for monitoring and management of pediatric patients during and after sedation for diagnostic and therapeutic procedures. *Pediatrics* **89**, 1110–1115.

CHAPTER 10

SPECIFIC PLANS FOR PAIN PREVENTION AND CONTROL

Neil S. Morton

Neonates and infants

Emergency surgery

Major surgery

Intensive care

Intermediate surgery

Day case surgery

Sedation for diagnostic and therapeutic procedures

Chronic medical conditions

Troubleshooting analgesic techniques

There is no single correct analgesic technique for each procedure but the following plans may be useful. Each plan must be adapted to the locally available facilities, personnel and training. The principles underlying these pain management plans are:

- use of the simplest effective technique
- a multimodal approach
- regular reassessment and titration of analgesia for each individual child

NEONATES AND INFANTS

Premature infants and formerly premature infants are at increased risk of post-operative apnoea, bradycardia and oxygen desaturation following a general anaesthetic. It is not certain whether post-operative apnoea is the consequence of the unmasking of immature respiratory control by residual general anaesthetic effects, post-operative pain, neurohumoral substances or other factors. Oxygen desaturation occurs owing to both central apnoea and obstructive apnoea. Therefore it is recommended that full term infants up to a post-conceptual age of 44 weeks should undergo apnoea and pulse oximetry monitoring for at least 12 hours after general anaesthesia while formerly premature infants up to 60 weeks post-conceptual age require monitoring in an HDU or ITU environment for a minimum of 24 hours after elective surgery regardless of the anaesthetic technique used. Pain management in this group of patients has to consider these specific risks. Pulse oximetry should be used when possible to detect hypoxaemia and chest wall impedance monitoring detects central apnoeas. Administration of supplemental oxygen does not eliminate the incidence of apnoea or oxygen desaturation and a small number of these infants will require active treatment for their oxygen desaturations. Therefore as preterm infants are more prone to complications following minor surgery than term infants their anaesthesia and analgesia should be undertaken by specifically trained personnel in hospitals with both adequate monitoring facilities and staffing levels. Access to intensive care beds is mandatory for these patients as any procedure, no matter how minor, may be life threatening. However, procedural pain can be reduced safely by analgesics, and major physiologic and behavioural disturbances can be prevented.

CAPILLARY BLOOD SAMPLING IN A NEONATE

- is this capillary sample necessary?
- is there an indwelling intravascular line to sample from?
- would venepuncture be less painful and technically easier?
- use comforting measures
- use automatic, spring-loaded heel lance
- use 'sucrose analgesia' and/or feed prior to sampling if possible
- consider amethocaine gel for topical anaesthesia

VENEPUNCTURE IN A NEONATE

- use topical local anaesthetic
- consider sucrose analgesia in neonates and small infants
- consider nitrous oxide/oxygen via conventional oxygen face mask
- consider ice or ethyl chloride spray
- use comfort and/or distraction measures, e.g. blowing bubbles, guided imagery
- use small needle
- give paracetamol

HERNIOTOMY IN A NEONATE

- in preterm or ex-preterm neonate, consider awake spinal +/− caudal (+/− caudal catheter) with topical local anaesthesia to all puncture sites and sucrose analgesia, paracetamol pre- and post-operative, early oral intake
- instillation or infiltration of wound with local

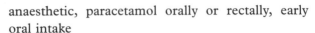
anaesthetic, paracetamol orally or rectally, early oral intake
- inguinal block or caudal, paracetamol, early oral intake
- if block fails, consider 5 micrograms/kg iv morphine increments titrated every 5 minutes or codeine phosphate 1 mg/kg im while still anaesthetized

CIRCUMCISION IN A NEONATE
- topical lignocaine gel to foreskin area, paracetamol
- penile block, topical lignocaine gel, paracetamol
- caudal, topical lignocaine gel, paracetamol
- in preterm or ex-preterm neonate awake spinal and/ or caudal with topical local anaesthesia to all puncture sites and sucrose analgesia, topical lignocaine gel, paracetamol, early oral intake

PYLOROMYOTOMY
- wound instillation or infiltration with local anaesthetic, paracetamol, early oral intake
- rectus sheath or paraumbilical block, paracetamol, early oral intake

LAPAROTOMY IN A NEONATE OR INFANT
- epidural via caudal catheter maintained by top-ups or continuous infusion for 24–36 hours (caution with dose; beware opioids if not ventilated), paracetamol, intensive care
- wound instillation or infiltration with local anaesthetic, fentanyl or alfentanil or remifentanil, paracetamol, intravenous morphine boluses 5 micrograms/kg repeated every 5 minutes to

desired effect or infusion 5–20 micrograms/kg/hr, intensive care area for post-operative care

- use higher doses of opioids if electively ventilating baby and add low dose sedative such as midazolam
- if stress control vital, consider spinal plus epidural in specialist centres only

THORACOTOMY IN A NEONATE OR INFANT

- intra-operative fentanyl, alfentanil, remifentanil, or low dose morphine, wound infiltration with local anaesthetic, consider iv morphine boluses 5 micrograms/kg repeated every 5 minutes to desired effect or infusion 5–20 micrograms/kg/hr, paracetamol, intensive care
- intra-operative opioid, intercostal nerve block, paracetamol
- paravertebral or interpleural catheter, paracetamol
- epidural via caudal catheter, paracetamol

CLEFT LIP AND PALATE REPAIR IN AN INFANT

- infra-orbital nerve block and local infiltration, paracetamol
- during anaesthesia if airway anatomy and maturity normal, consider codeine phosphate, 1 mg/kg im or morphine increments of 20 micrograms/kg iv, repeated up to 100 micrograms/kg
- in recovery, titrate morphine 5 micrograms/kg increments every 5 minutes if distressed, consider iv morphine infusion up to 20 micrograms/kg/hr
- consider diclofenac 1 mg/kg rectally in older infants
- for alveolar bone graft, consider bupivacaine wound perfusion of iliac crest donor site

EMERGENCY SURGERY

LACERATION REPAIR

- instillation or topical application of local anaesthetic and vasoconstrictor (e.g. bupivacaine/noradrenaline), infiltration of local anaesthetic, distraction or guided imagery, paracetamol and/or NSAIDs
- digital or metacarpal block, paracetamol and/or NSAIDs
- entonox, local infiltration or block, paracetamol and/or NSAIDs
- consider sedation or general anaesthesia with local anaesthesia technique and paracetamol and/or NSAIDs

APPENDICECTOMY

- iv morphine, wound infiltration, paracetamol and/or NSAIDs, iv morphine boluses, infusion or PCA
- iv morphine, intercostal nerve block, paracetamol and/or NSAIDs, iv morphine boluses, infusion or PCA

LAPAROTOMY

- iv morphine, wound infiltration, paracetamol and/or NSAIDs, iv morphine boluses, infusion or PCA
- epidural local anaesthetic by top-up or continuous infusion +/− opioid, paracetamol, rescue iv morphine

FRACTURES

- iv morphine titrated to comfort up to 0.2 mg/kg, paracetamol and/or NSAIDs
- nitrous oxide, haematoma block or digital or metacarpal or metatarsal block

- femoral nerve block by single injection or catheter technique or 3–in-1 block
- iv regional anaesthesia (Bier's block)
- consider sedation or general anaesthesia with plexus block or caudal block or continuous epidural catheter technique for major injuries
- consider iv morphine boluses, infusion, PCA, or subcutaneous morphine plus paracetamol and/or NSAIDs, low dose diazepam for skeletal muscle spasm prevention

HEAD INJURY

- local anaesthesia to surface lacerations
- if conscious level normal and in severe pain, titrate small doses of iv morphine 20 micrograms/kg to achieve analgesia
- for moderate pain give paracetamol/codeine combination or dihydrocodeine

BURNS

- iv morphine titrated to achieve adequate analgesia, then iv infusion or PCA or NCA, paracetamol
- consider oral sustained release morphine for maintenance analgesia
- consider benzodiazepines for anxiolysis and background sedation and amnesia
- consider antihistamine for itching (low dose iv lignocaine infusion may be useful for this symptom if severe and patient is fully monitored in HDU or ICU area)

BURNS DRESSINGS

- consider general anaesthesia or anaesthetist supervised anaesthesia with midazolam/fentanyl or propofol or ketamine

- ensure adequate monitoring and supervision of child during procedure
- oral midazolam premedication is helpful, extra bolus doses of morphine prior to procedure by nurse or patient if on PCA
- consider nitrous oxide
- use non-drug methods, e.g. music, distraction, imagery, relaxation
- local anaesthesia to donor site: nerve block or soak donor site dressing, maintain with dressing perfusion technique

MAJOR SURGERY

ANTERIOR SPINAL FUSION
- iv morphine, infusion or PCA, paracetamol, NSAIDs added after 24 hours
- epidural infusion or top-ups with paracetamol, NSAIDs after 24 hours

POSTERIOR SPINAL FUSION
- iv morphine or fentanyl then morphine infusion or PCA and paracetamol, add NSAIDs from day 2 onwards

LEG LENGTHENING AND OSTEOTOMIES
- epidural top-ups or infusion
- plexus block or single shot caudal block, iv or sc morphine bolus, infusion or PCA, paracetamol, NSAIDs, low dose diazepam for muscle spasms

CARDIAC SURGERY
- intraoperative high dose opioid then iv morphine infusion or PCA, with paracetamol and NSAIDs after 24 hours

Thoracic surgery
- wound infiltration or intercostal nerve blocks, intra-operative opioid then iv morphine infusion or PCA, with paracetamol and NSAIDs after 24 hours
- thoracic epidural
- paravertebral catheter, paracetamol, NSAIDs
- consider nitrous oxide and local anaesthetic infiltration for chest drain removal

INTENSIVE CARE

- iv morphine infusion, midazolam, paracetamol
- NCA morphine
- local anaesthesia as appropriate
- consider fentanyl, alfentanil, remifentanil for special indications

INTERMEDIATE SURGERY

Adenotonsillectomy
- paracetamol premedication, iv morphine intra-operative and early post-operative, paracetamol +/− NSAIDs, antiemetic cover (ondansetron, trimeprazine)
- avoid local anaesthetic infiltration (ineffective, high peak plasma concentrations)
- consider paracetamol/codeine combination for older children

Hypospadias correction
- single shot caudal +/− additives (opioid or clonidine or ketamine), morphine iv or sc boluses, infusion or PCA, paracetamol +/− NSAIDs

233

- consider low dose diazepam or oxybutyline for bladder spasms
- consider continuous epidural technique for more complex repairs, give benzodiazepine for mild sedation and anxiolysis

URETERIC REIMPLANTATION
- wound infiltration, iv morphine boluses, infusion or PCA, paracetamol, NSAIDs if renal function normal
- single shot caudal +/− additives, morphine, paracetamol, NSAIDs as above
- continuous epidural technique

PYELOPLASTY
- wound infiltration or intercostal nerve blocks (T6–T12), iv morphine boluses, infusion or PCA, paracetamol, NSAIDs if renal function normal
- continuous thoracic epidural with catheter tip at T9, paracetamol, rescue morphine
- consider low dose benzodiazepine for sedation, anxiolysis and antispasmodic effects

DAY CASE SURGERY

HERNIOTOMY, HYDROCELE, ORCHIDOPEXY
- instillation or infiltration of wound with local anaesthetic or inguinal block or caudal, paracetamol +/− NSAIDs orally or rectally, early oral intake, may need antiemetic for orchidopexy
- if block fails, consider 20 micrograms/kg iv morphine increments

CIRCUMCISION
- topical lignocaine gel to foreskin area, paracetamol
- penile block, topical lignocaine gel, paracetamol
- caudal, topical lignocaine gel, paracetamol

UMBILICAL HERNIA REPAIR
- wound instillation or infiltration, paracetamol +/− NSAIDs
- consider rectus sheath or paraumbilical block, paracetamol +/− NSAIDs

SQUINT CORRECTION
- topical local anaesthetic eye drops (amethocaine or oxybuprocaine), paracetamol +/− NSAIDs
- topical NSAID eye drops (diclofenac, ketorolac), paracetamol +/− NSAIDs
- avoid opioids except as rescue analgesia

MYRINGOTOMY
- paracetamol +/− NSAIDs

SEDATION FOR DIAGNOSTIC AND THERAPEUTIC PROCEDURES

BONE MARROW SAMPLING AND LUMBAR PUNCTURE
- topical local anaesthesia to all puncture sites
- oral midazolam premedication
- nitrous oxide
- midazolam supplements
- iv morphine increments
- consider general anaesthesia, e.g. with propofol or ketamine or both

RENAL BIOPSY
- topical local anaesthesia to all puncture sites
- oral midazolam premedication
- nitrous oxide
- midazolam supplements
- iv morphine increments
- consider general anaesthesia, e.g. with propofol or ketamine or both

CT OR MRI SCAN
- oral midazolam premedication
- midazolam supplements
- consider general anaesthesia

CARDIAC CATHETERIZATION
- topical local anaesthesia to all puncture sites
- oral midazolam premedication
- midazolam supplements
- consider general anaesthesia

CHRONIC MEDICAL CONDITIONS

CANCER PAIN
Cancer pain may be due to the disease or to treatment. Pain may come from invasion of bone, nerves or local rapid expansion of a tumour mass. Bowel or urinary tract obstruction may cause colicky discomfort. Headache owing to raised intracranial pressure or bony invasion may be severe and associated with nausea and vomiting. Back pain may be due to bone invasion, spinal cord or nerve root invasion or compression and protective muscle spasm. Pain owing to treatment may be from needling procedures, infections, mucositis, radiation injury to bowel, bladder or bone, peripheral

neuropathy or neuropathic pain. Management of cancer pain relies on an accurate diagnosis and good planning with detailed attention to both the emotional and physical components of pain (**Boxes 10.1–10.3**).

The World Health Organisation pain control ladder is a useful approach with stepwise increases in potency of analgesics to match the severity of pain (**Figure 10.1**).

SICKLE CELL DISEASE

The pain in sickle cell disease is due to occlusion of capillaries by sickled red cells which causes ischaemia of bone, gut and other organs. Pain is intermittent, severe and recurrent. A planned stepwise approach to pain control with early intervention at home to prevent progression to severe pain is essential and it is helpful to have an individualized set of written instructions for each child and family to follow. At home, encouraging regular fluid intake to prevent dehydration is important and staying warm and well clad in cold weather is a

---

An approach to cancer pain in children

- assess the site, nature, severity and timing of pain along with factors that make it better or worse
- construct an individual pain management plan for each child using drug and non-drug methods to control pain and to treat the disease
- ensure involvement of child and parents in sharing the assessment and control procedures
- use the WHO pain control ladder
- pay attention to identification and management of other symptoms (see **Box 10.2**)

Box 10.1

Symptom control in children with cancer

- inflammatory or bone pain: NSAIDs
- oedema reduction: steroids
- mass reduction: radiotherapy
- gastrointestinal pain: loperamide or hyoscine
- headaches: steroids, intrathecal chemotherapy
- breathlessness: opioids, benzodiazepines, oxygen therapy
- cough: inhalations of menthol
- secretions: hyoscine
- insomnia: deal with fears, benzodiazepines
- neuropathic pain: tricyclics, anticonvulsants, nerve blocks, TENS
- muscle spasms: diazepam, baclofen
- altered or interrupted sleep: pain control, benzodiazepines, antidepressants, antihallucinogens (e.g. haloperidol)

Box 10.2

simple preventative measure. Management of mild pain should be started early with regular on-the-clock 4 hourly paracetamol, supplemented by an NSAID and oral codeine given regularly if pain is moderate and oral morphine for severe pain. If pain is not controlled in 12 hours, is not of the usual character, is accompanied by a fever of 38°C or more and especially if nausea and vomiting prevent adequate dosing with oral medication, help should be sought at hospital. For severe pain in hospital, intravenous morphine is titrated to gain pain control. Maintenance of pain control may require very large hourly morphine doses and patient-controlled analgesia with morphine is very useful in the acute stage to accommodate the wide variation between patients. Oxygen therapy and pulse oximetry monitoring are started and intravenous fluids may be needed. For severe lower limb pain, epidural analgesia may be

▼

Doses of drugs used for symptom control in cancer in children

- amitriptyline 0.5–1.5 mg/kg orally once in the evening
- baclofen 1 mg/kg/day in three divided doses
- carbamazepine 2.5 mg/kg bd, gradually increasing to 5–10 mg/kg bd
- codeine 0.5–1 mg/kg orally up to every 4 hours
- dexamethasone 0.1 mg/kg/day oral/iv; high dose regimen 0.25–1 mg/kg/day in divided doses
- diamorphine 0.05 mg/kg iv then titrated infusion iv or sc
- diazepam 0.1–0.2 mg/kg up to every 6 hours
- diclofenac 1 mg/kg up to every 8 hours
- haloperidol 0.025–0.1 mg/kg/day
- hyoscine butylbromide for GI pain 5–10 mg up to every 8 hours
- hyoscine hydrobromide for secretions 10 micrograms/kg up to every 6 hours
- ibuprofen 10 mg/kg up to every 6 hours
- ketorolac 0.5 mg/kg up to every 6 hours
- loperamide 25–50 micrograms/kg up to every 6 hours
- methadone start at 0.2 mg/kg up to every 12 hours
- midazolam 0.05–0.2 mg/kg iv, 0.5 mg/kg oral, iv or sc infusion titrated as required in terminal care
- morphine 0.1 mg/kg iv bolus, iv or sc infusion titrated to effect, PCA as in text; oral immediate release 1–2 mg/kg/24 hours in six divided doses; oral controlled release morphine 1 mg/kg every 12 hours with 1–2 mg/kg immediate release morphine for breakthrough pain; review total daily morphine consumption and prescribe this for next 24 hours
- naproxen 5 mg/kg every 12 hours
- paracetamol 15–20 mg/kg orally every 4 hours; 20–30 mg/kg rectally every 6 hours
- temazepam 0.5–1 mg/kg in evening
- tramadol 1–2 mg/kg up to every 6 hours

Box 10.3

beneficial. Heat therapy, TENS, hypnosis, distraction and coping techniques can all be helpful in individual cases. Stepwise weaning as pain declines should be carried out slowly over several days.

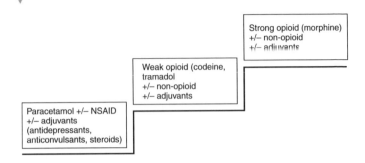

Figure 10.1
WHO pain control ladder

COMPLEX CHRONIC PAIN SYNDROMES

The names of chronic pain syndromes have changed recently because terms such as reflex sympathetic dystrophy are not always accurate. They are now classified as complex regional pain syndrome (CRPS) types 1 and 2 depending on whether there is an identifiable nerve lesion present or not. CRPS type 1 is seen in children and often develops after a relatively minor injury and manifests as ongoing pain which is more widespread and severe than would be expected from the initial injury and may be exacerbated by non-noxious stimuli. There is increased sensitivity to noxious and non-noxious stimuli and variable degrees of swelling, bruising, sweating and changes in temperature and skin blood flow. Sometimes, dystrophic changes are seen in the skin and wasting of muscles may occur. Diagnosis is helped by radiology, thermal imaging, and response to trials of sympathetic blockade. Treatment is with physiotherapy, sympathetic blockade, sympatholytic agents, tricyclics and anticonvulsants. Other agents such as clonidine, adenosine, steroids, NSAIDs and TENS may help individual cases. Coping strategies and encouragement back towards normal function, activity level, schooling and family life are vital for success. Results are much improved if the condition is recognized and treated aggressively at an early stage.

JUVENILE RHEUMATOID ARTHRITIS

Management of pain, inflammation, mobility and psychological factors are all relevant. An analgesic ladder approach is appropriate with more emphasis on large doses of paracetamol, NSAIDs and salicylates and less on opioids. Steroids, immunosuppressants and long acting agents such as penicillamine all have a role but the management must be coordinated by a rheumatology specialist. Behavioural therapy and coping strategies are essential for child and family and considerable close follow-up and support will be needed for these families.

TROUBLESHOOTING ANALGESIC TECHNIQUES

BREAKTHROUGH PAIN

- firstly assess the patient: diagnose site, severity and cause of the pain
- if receiving a continuous morphine infusion, give the last hour's dose as a bolus +/− increase infusion rate by up to 50%; review increase after 1 hour
- if on PCA, check equipment, delivery pathway, patient's ability to use device; increase bolus dose by up to 50%, check lockout interval 5 minutes, consider concurrent analgesic prescription with NSAID and paracetamol and ensure patient is actually getting these
- is there a technical problem with an epidural, is an alternative analgesic technique more appropriate?

- would patient benefit from anxiolytic, antispasmodic or night sedative to restore sleep pattern?
- does the pain or distress respond to comforting, cognitive or behavioural measures?

RESPIRATORY DEPRESSION

- if very sedated, SpO_2 <90%, slow respiratory rate and bradycardia, start ABC of resuscitation (Airway, Breathing, Circulation), switch off opioid, give oxygen, give naloxone 2 micrograms/kg repeated as required up to 10 micrograms/kg then infusion of 10 micrograms/kg/hr

NAUSEA AND VOMITING

- use opioid sparing techniques
- give ondansetron 0.1 mg/kg iv, repeated up to every 6 hours
- check for surgical or medical causes, e.g. ileus, bowel obstruction

CONSTIPATION

- check cause, discuss with surgeons
- use opioid sparing techniques
- suppositories, enemas, stool softeners, laxatives

URINARY RETENTION

- opioid sparing techniques
- prophylactic catheterization if continuous epidural technique planned, especially if with mixture of local anaesthetic and opioid
- naloxone 0.5–2 micrograms/kg may work
- suprapubic expression of bladder possible in younger children

ITCHING

- consider cause
- chlorpheniramine 0.1 mg/kg orally or slow iv may be useful but produces significant sedation and enhances opioid-induced sedation
- naloxone in low dose 0.5 micrograms/kg may help
- ondansetron 0.1 mg/kg orally or iv may be useful for itching due to epidural or intrathecal opioids

MUSCLE SPASMS

- continuous epidural or block techniques are most effective for skeletal muscle spasms in orthopaedic patients
- diazepam 0.1 mg/kg every 6 hours is useful for both skeletal and visceral muscle spasms, e.g. after hypospadias repair, renal tract surgery
- oxybutyline is useful for bladder spasms 5 mg every 8–12 hours

RESTLESSNESS/TWITCHING

- seen in infants receiving continuous opioids ('morphine jerks'): may be due to accumulation of stimulatory metabolites such as M3G or norpethidine, responds to reducing opioid infusion rate
- may be a sign of local anaesthetic toxicity: check dose, pump function and delivery pathway; consider reducing dose
- may respond to low dose benzodiazepine especially for night sedation if neither of above apply

KEY LEARNING POINTS

- careful selection and tailoring of analgesia can allow pain free return to function in the majority of children which helps to minimize the psychological upset and prevents chronic pain
- a choice of analgesic methods is usually available and it is good practice to use the simplest effective method as this will usually be safest
- identification and management of inadequate analgesia and adverse effects is vital
- long term pain in childhood requires a multidisciplinary, structured approach

FURTHER READING

Aynsley-Green A., Ward Platt M.P. and Lloyd-Thomas A.R. (1995) Stress and pain in infancy and childhood. *Bailliere's Clinical Paediatrics* **3**, 449–631.

Howard R.F. (1996) Planning for pain relief. *Bailliere's Clinical Anaesthesiology* **10**, 657–675.

Macintyre P.E. and Ready L.B. (1996) *Acute Pain Management: A Practical Guide.* WB Saunders, London.

Royal College of Paediatrics and Child Health (1997) *Prevention and Control of Pain in Children.* BMJ Publishing Group, London.

Stevens B. (1996) Management of painful procedures in the newborn. *Current Opinion in Paediatrics* **8**, 102–107.

APPENDIX I

PRACTICAL PAIN ASSESSMENT TOOLS

• FACES SCALE

• VERTICAL VISUAL
  ANALOGUE RULER

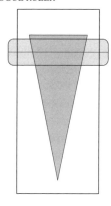 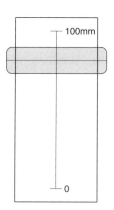

100mm

0

• POKER CHIP TOOL
  ('PIECES OF HURT')

APPENDIX 2

EXAMPLE OF A PAEDIATRIC
ACUTE PAIN RELIEF SERVICE
(APRS) PROTOCOL

Minimum monitoring standard
One nurse per 4 patients; continuous pulse oximetry; hourly nurse recordings using appropriate monitoring charts; twice daily visits by pain relief nurse specialist and duty anaesthetists; once daily visit by pain consultant.

General points
Doses are a guide only and should be titrated against monitoring results. The medical condition, surgical condition, age and maturity of the child will affect the regimen. Refilling of opioid syringes should be performed by ward medical staff after appropriate training. Programming or reprogramming of PCA devices should only be performed by the APRS. Refilling local anaesthetic syringes and epidural top-ups should only be performed by anaesthetic staff. Ensure all syringes for opioid or local anaesthetic infusions are correctly labelled using the red additive labels. Ensure prescription is correctly and legibly written, signed, dated and timed on the additive label, in the drug Kardex and on the monitoring chart. Ensure the appropriate monitoring chart has all the requested information accurately filled in and accompanies the patient to the ward or PICU.

Beware!
Double check: drug dosages, drug dilutions, pump settings, concurrent prescription of different opioids,

actual or potentially poor peripheral perfusion when the SC route is used, gravity free flow/siphonage/reflux of opioids, injection or infusion of the wrong substance into epidurals.

OPIOID INFUSIONS

Loading doses
Consider loading dose of morphine if >3 months old; 0.1–0.2 mg/kg, i.e. 100–200 micrograms/kg; omit if <3 months or has good local/regional block or has received another opioid.

Intravenous morphine (IVM) infusion
Use dedicated cannula or anti-free flow plus antireflux valve.

Morphine 1 mg/kg in 50 ml 0.9% saline ($\equiv$ 0.02 mg/kg/ml, i.e. 20 micrograms/kg/ml); maximum 50 mg in 50 ml

Age 0–1 months: up to 0.004 mg/kg/hr, i.e. 4 micrograms/kg/hr $\equiv$ 0.2 ml/hr
  >1–3 months: up to 0.010 mg/kg/hr, i.e. 10 micrograms/kg/hr $\equiv$ 0.5 ml/hr
  >3 months: up to 0.020 mg/kg/hr, i.e. 20 micrograms/kg/hr $\equiv$ 1.0 ml/hr [may need up to 2.0 ml/hr]

Intravenous patient-controlled analgesia with morphine (IVPCAM)
Use dedicated cannula or anti-free flow plus antireflux valve.

Morphine 1 mg/kg in 50 ml 0.9% saline ($\equiv$ 0.02 mg/kg/ml, i.e. 20 micrograms/kg/ml); maximum 50 mg in 50 ml

Initial IVPCAM settings for paediatrics

Bolus dose 0.020 mg/kg, i.e. 20 micrograms/kg $\equiv$ 1.0 ml; maximum bolus dose 1 mg

Lockout interval 5 minutes

Background infusion 0.004 mg/kg/hr, i.e. 4 micrograms/kg/hr $\equiv$ 0.2 ml/hr [especially first 24 hr]

Subcutaneous patient-controlled analgesia with morphine (SCPCAM)

Use 24G cannula over deltoid or anterior abdominal wall.

Morphine 1 mg/kg in 20 ml 0.9% saline ($\equiv$ 0.05 mg/kg/ml, i.e. 50 micrograms/kg/ml); maximum 50 mg in 20 ml

Initial SCPCAM settings for paediatrics

Bolus dose 0.020 mg/kg, i.e. 20 micrograms/kg $\equiv$ 0.4 ml; maximum bolus dose 1 mg

Lockout interval 5 minutes

Background infusion 0.005 mg/kg/hr, i.e. 5 micrograms/kg/hr $\equiv$ 0.1 ml/hr [especially first 24 hr]

Subcutaneous morphine infusion (SCM)

Use 24G cannula over deltoid or anterior abdominal wall.

Morphine 1 mg/kg in 20 ml 0.9% saline ($\equiv$ 0.05 mg/kg/ml, i.e. 50 micrograms/kg/ml); maximum 50 mg in 20 ml

Age 0–1 months: up to 0.005 mg/kg/hr, i.e. 5 micrograms/kg/hr $\equiv$ 0.1 ml/hr

>1–3 months: up to 0.010 mg/kg/hr, i.e. 10 micrograms/kg/hr $\equiv$ 0.2 ml/hr

>3 months: up to 0.020 mg/kg/hr, i.e. 20 micrograms/kg/hr $\equiv$ 0.4 ml/hr [may need up to 0.6 ml/hr]

CO-ANALGESIA

Paracetamol 20 mg/kg loading dose, then 15 mg/kg up to 4 hourly oral/pr [time doses for first 48 hr]; maximum dose in 24 hr 90 mg/kg. *Caution if liver dysfunction.*

Diclofenac 1 mg/kg up to 8 hourly o/pr [time doses for first 48 hr]. *Caution if bleeding risk, asthma, atopy, renal dysfunction, GI ulceration/bleeding, on anticoagulants.*

Ibuprofen 10 mg/kg up to 6 hourly oral [time doses for first 48 hr]. *Caution if bleeding risk, asthma, atopy, renal dysfunction, GI ulceration/bleeding, on anticoagulants.*

WEANING FROM COMPLEX ANALGESIA

Ensure adequate doses of co-analgesics are prescribed and are being given to achieve morphine-sparing effect; wean down infusion rate depending on monitoring results; liaise with surgical colleagues about oral intake, rectal route for drugs, mobilization, dressings, drain/catheter removal. If prolonged opioid use, wean slowly (20% per day) to avoid withdrawal syndrome. For specific cases consider step across analgesia with dihydrocodeine, 0.5–1 mg/kg orally 6 hourly or tramadol, 1–2 mg/kg orally/iv/pr provided morphine has been stopped *(avoid concurrent prescription of opioids).*

EPIDURAL BUPIVACAINE (PLAIN SOLUTIONS)

In theatre

<8 years 0.25% bupivacaine up to 1.0 ml/kg in fractionated doses (may need less for thoracic epidural).

8 years + 0.5% bupivacaine up to 0.5 ml/kg in fractionated doses (may need less for thoracic epidural).

If 6 months+ place SC cannula for rescue analgesia

and prescribe 0.1 mg/kg sc morphine which can be given by ward nursing staff.

If <6 months use IV route for rescue analgesia and prescribe 0.01–0.05 mg/kg (10–50 micrograms/kg) iv morphine given by ward doctor.

In recovery

Check block, check adequacy of analgesia, check adequacy of sedation, check for restlessness.

Top up if required with 0.25% bupivacaine.

If restless, < 6 months give iv morphine 0.01–0.05 mg/kg
(10–50 micrograms/kg)
6 months+ give sc morphine 0.1 mg/kg

If epidural is not working after top-ups and partial withdrawal of catheter, take it out and change to another form of analgesia.

Post-operative

Either

Top-up regimen

<8 years bupivacaine 0.25% 0.1–0.3 ml/kg in fractionated doses (may need less for thoracic epidural).

8 years+ bupivacaine 0.375% 0.1–0.2 ml/kg in fractionated doses (may need less for thoracic epidural).

Top-ups usually last for 4–12 hours in children. Check block; give top-up in fractionated doses; check BP, HR, RR, SpO_2 every 5 minutes for 15 minutes; recheck block and pain score.

Or

Infusion regimen

<6 months bupivacaine infusion 0.125% plain @ 0.2–0.3 ml/kg/hr ≡ 0.25–0.375 mg/kg/hr

May need top-ups 0.25% bupivacaine 0.1–0.3 ml/kg ≡ 0.25–0.75 mg/kg in fractionated doses [maximum total dose (including top-ups) per 4 hr period 1.5 mg/kg]

6 months+ bupivacaine infusion 0.125% plain @ 0.2–0.4 ml/kg/hr ≡ 0.25–0.5 mg/kg/hr

May need top-ups 0.25% bupivacaine 0.1–0.3 ml/kg ≡ 0.25–0.75 mg/kg in fractionated doses [maximum total dose (including top-ups) per 4 hr period 2.0 mg/kg]

Consider bupivacaine 0.125% + morphine or fentanyl (see Box 6.12, page 166)

Rescue analgesia

If 6 months+ place SC cannula for rescue analgesia and prescribe 0.1 mg/kg sc morphine which can be given by ward nursing staff or ward doctor. If no sc cannula, iv morphine 0.1 mg/kg can be given by ward doctor, anaesthetist or certificated nurse.

If <6 months use IV route for rescue analgesia and prescribe 0.01–0.05 mg/kg (10–50 micrograms/kg) iv morphine given by ward doctor.

Do not give parenteral opioids if receiving epidural opioids.

Antagonists

Naloxone 2–10 micrograms/kg iv stat; can be repeated every 60 seconds or start infusion at 10 micrograms/kg/hr; use lowest effective dose; if no venous access give im 100 micrograms/kg

Flumazenil 5 micrograms/kg iv stat; can be repeated every 60 seconds or start infusion at 10 micrograms/kg/hr

Antiemetics
Ondansetron 0.1 mg/kg iv or oral; droperidol 0.01–0.05 mg/kg iv or 0.25 mg/kg oral; trimeprazine 0.25 mg/kg oral; transdermal hyoscine patch.

Muscle spasms in orthopaedics/bladder spasms in urology
Diazepam 0.1 mg/kg 6 hourly oral.

Dressing and drain removals
Consider Entonox (use Entonox protocol), opioid bolus, epidural top-up.

Skin graft donor sites
Lyofoam dressing soaked with 2 mg/kg bupivacaine 0.25% plain/1:200,000 adrenaline; put epidural catheter on dressing surface and infuse 0.25% bupivacaine at 0.1–0.2 ml/kg/hr $\equiv$ 0.25–0.5 mg/kg/hr; use wound perfusion monitoring chart.

Bone graft donor sites
Wound perfusion with bupivacaine 0.25% plain @ 0.1 ml/kg/hr $\equiv$ 0.25 mg/kg/hr; use wound perfusion monitoring chart.

APPENDIX 3

EXAMPLE OF PARENTAL
INFORMATION PCA

WHAT IS PCA?

PCA is short for Patient-Controlled Analgesia – the patient administers his or her own pain killing medicine using a hand-held button that is connected to a computerized pump.

WHAT THE SYSTEM CONSISTS OF:

A syringe filled with a pain killing drug such as morphine is fitted into the PCA pump. This is connected to a small plastic tube in the hand or arm. A button which is held in your child's hand is pushed by your child when he or she feels uncomfortable or sore. This will tell the pump to deliver a dose of the pain killing medicine.

HOW THE SYSTEM WORKS:

The pump is programmed in the recovery area by the anaesthetist after your child has had their operation. The anaesthetist will work out the suitable dose for your child taking into account their weight and age. On return to the ward the pump cannot be altered without discussion with the Pain Relief Team. Your child cannot be overdosed with the medicine as there is a safety device called a 'lockout' time. This is a period of time after your child has received a dose of medicine when the machine will not deliver another dose – even if the button is pressed.

OBSERVING YOUR CHILD USING PCA:

The nurses in the ward will watch your child closely when they are using PCA. They will check the pump hourly to see how many times your child is using the pump, to assess if he or she is using it properly and a pain score is recorded at each observation – usually hourly. The nursing staff will encourage your child to press the button and you should also encourage them if you feel he or she is starting to become uncomfortable.

If your child is to have physiotherapy, get out of bed for the first time since their operation or do anything that may cause discomfort, the nurses will ask your child to press the button 10–15 minutes beforehand, so he or she can feel more comfortable during the procedure.

WHAT AGE OF CHILD CAN USE PCA?

Children who are suitable for using PCA are identified by the anaesthetists before they have their operation. The child must

(a) have the physical ability to push the button of the handset.
(b) have a basic understanding of what happens when the button is pushed.

The patient is the only person who should press the pump; if he or she cannot manage to do so or cannot understand the idea of PCA, he or she should have another form of pain relief. It will not help the child if someone else is pressing the button for them and may be harmful.

I hope this answers any queries you may have about PCA but if there is anything else that you would like to discuss, please ask to speak to the Nurse Specialist, Pain Relief.

Contact Clinical Nurse Specialist, Pain Relief: Page 2133/ext. 0449. Any problems: Monday to Friday: 0830 1700

PCA Protocol

(Please place completed chart in casenotes)

Name.................................Unit No.............D.o.B...............Age............Weight.............

Operation...Date...

Morphine Concn. (1mg/kg in 50 mls 0.9% Saline ie 0.02mg/kg/ml) = ...mg/ml (maximum 50mg in 50mls)

Bolus dose (0.02mg/kg) = ...mg (= 1ml)

Lockout interval 5 min. Background infusion 0.2ml/hr (0.004mg/kg/hr) = ...mg/hr

Any adjustments (specify type, reason and time made)...

Serial No. of Pump ....

Signature of Anaesthetist ....

Date & time commenced ....

Record hourly

Time	SpO$_2$	Resp Rate	Sedation Score Eyes open: 0 = Spontaneously 1 = To speech 2 = To shake	Pain score at rest 0 = No pain A = Asleep 1 = Not really sore 2 = Quite sore	Pain score on movement (deep breath in and cough)	Nausea Score 0 = None 1 = Nausea only 2 = Vomiting ×1 in last hour	Total dose since reset	Number of presses and % good	Volume left in syringe

3 = Unrousable (Call Doctor)	3 = Very sore (Crying) (Call Doctor)	3 = Vomiting >1 in last hour (Call Doctor)	(press verify)

CALL DOCTOR if severe pain (score 3), patient unrousable (sedation score 3), SpO_2 <90. Respiration rate less than 10 if over 5 years, less than 20 if under 5 years, excessive nausea or vomiting, drip blocked/tissued or pump alarming. If patient unrousable, switch pump off and consider naloxone 10 micrograms/kg IV

CONTACT duty anaesthetist bleep 2602 if help needed, or Dr...............................Home no................

257

APPENDIX 5

EXAMPLE OF PARENTAL
INFORMATION: EPIDURALS

WHAT IS AN EPIDURAL?

This is an extremely effective method of pain relief. It takes the form of a very fine tube being introduced into your child's back when they are asleep from the anaesthetic. The tube is placed in an area called the 'epidural space'. This space contains nerves that send messages to your child's brain when they are in pain. The tube is introduced into your child's back by a needle. The needle is then pulled out leaving the tube in place. There will be sticky tape on your child's back to stop the tube falling out. Local anaesthetic is given through the tube to 'block' these nerves and stop the pain messages being carried. This means that the area of the surgery is numb and less painful.

HOW IS THE LOCAL ANAESTHETIC GIVEN?

There are two ways that we give our local anaesthetic medicine in this hospital. The first is that your child may have a computerized pump attached to the tube in his or her back. The pump is programmed by the anaesthetist to give a suitable dose of the local anaesthetic to your child continuously via the tube. The other method is that your child will receive the medicine only when they start to feel sore. This is called a 'top up'. The anaesthetist will come and give them the medicine by using a syringe and squeezing it in slowly. The medicine may make your child's legs feel heavy and slightly numb – but don't worry, this is normal.

OBSERVING YOUR CHILD WITH AN EPIDURAL:

The nurses in the ward will observe your child closely when they have an epidural. They will check hourly to see if your child is comfortable and that the epidural is working properly. They will check the blood pressure as sometimes an epidural can lower it slightly.

If your child is having the 'top up' method, the nurses will check the blood pressure every five minutes for fifteen minutes after the top up is given. Your child will be lying down at this time so the medicine is spread equally and the right area is covered. Your child will be seen two or three times a day by the Pain Relief Service to make sure that they are comfortable.

OTHER POINTS:

If your child has the 'top up' version of the epidural method of pain relief, the medicine given can last any time from four hours to twelve hours. At night there is always an anaesthetist in the hospital 'on call'. It is their specialist job to look after the epidurals. However, they also have to be available for any emergency operations that have to take place. If your child starts to feel sore and the anaesthetist is in theatre, he may not be able to come to 'top up' your child straight away. To meet this problem, your child will have a small plastic tube called a cannula put in their arm when they are in theatre. He or she will not feel this and it will be held in place by a small piece of tape. Through this tube the nurses can give some strong pain killing medicine (usually morphine). This will stop your child feeling sore until the anaesthetist is able to come to the ward.

Before your child's epidural is stopped, he or she will be started on other pain killing medicine. This will usually take the form of syrup, tablets or suppositories that will be given regularly through the day.

I hope this answers any queries you may have about epidurals but if there is anything you would like to discuss, please ask to speak to the Nurse Specialist Pain Relief.

APPENDIX 6

Contact Clinical Nurse Specialist, Pain Relief: Page 2133/ext. 0449. Any problems: Monday to Friday: 0830 1700

Epidural Protocol

Serial No. of Pump....................

Signature of Anaesthetist....................

Date & time commenced....................

Name........................Unit No..........D.o.B..........Age..........Weight..........

Operation..........................Date..........

Epidural site	Thoracic	Lumbar	Caudal	1	2	3	4	5	6	7	8	9	10	11	12
Needle size	16G	18G	19G												

Length of Catheter in Epidural Space   cm   Mark on skin   cm

Prescription

In theatre	Bupivacaine	0.5%	0.25%	0.125%	0.166%	vol ml
In Recovery	Bupivacaine	0.5%	0.25%	0.125%	0.166%	vol ml
Infusion	Bupivacaine	0.125%	0.166%	AT _____ to _____ ml/hr
Top ups	Bupivacaine	0.25%	_____ mls

Max dosage per 4 hour period 1.25 - 1.5 mg/kg if < 6m; 2 mg/kg if ≥ 6m = [____] **mg per 4 hours**

Record hourly (AFTER TOP-UPS record every 5mins for 15mins)

Time	SpO₂	RR	BP sys/dia	HR	Height of Block	SEDATION SCORE Eyes open : 0 = Spontaneously = To speech 2 = To shake	PAIN SCORE at rest Eyes open: 0 = No pain A = Asleep 1 = Not really sore	NAUSEA SCORE 0 = None 1 = Nausea only 2 = Vomiting x1 in last hour 3 = **Vomiting**	RESTLESSNESS SCORE 0 = None 1 = Slight (easily calmed) 2 = Moderate	RECORD TOP-UPS as volume conc time or sedation as drug, mg, route, time	Volume left in syringe (mls)

3 = Unrousable (Call Doctor)	2 = Quite sore / 3 = Very sore (Crying) (Call Doctor)	>1 in last hour (Call Doctor)	(not easily calmed) 3 = Severe inconsolable may need top up sedation (call Doctor)		

CALL DOCTOR if pain score 3, nausea score 3; restlessness score 3:Syringe empty

CONTACT DOCTOR AND SWITCH OFF EPIDURAL if patient unrousable (score 3);SpO_2<90%

block height above [ ] ; HR< [ ] ;BP< [ ]

CONTACT duty anaesthetist bleep 2602 if help needed, or Dr...................................Home no.................

APPENDIX 7

EXAMPLE OF PARENTAL
INFORMATION: MORPHINE

Questions and concerns about pain medicines are normal. This handout contains information that will hopefully answer these questions about your child's pain relief. The medicines we use are safe and very effective and will help your child recover more easily and quickly from their surgery. If you have any more questions that are not answered in this handout please ask to speak to the Clinical Nurse Specialist in Pain Relief.

SOME COMMONLY ASKED QUESTIONS

Is morphine too strong for children?
Will my child become addicted to morphine?
Will my child experience unpleasant side effects from morphine?

WHY DO WE USE MORPHINE?

Your child may experience some pain after certain surgical procedures. Morphine or a morphine-like medication are some of the most effective medicines available to control this pain. These medicines are very safe when used properly. Your child should be able to move or cough without discomfort. If your child is to have physiotherapy after surgery and has good pain control the treatment will be much more effective. Recovery and healing should take place more quickly.

IS MORPHINE TOO STRONG?

The pain relief effects of morphine depend on the dose given. In this hospital the doses are worked out for the child by weight and age. The children are monitored carefully by the nurses and doctors in the wards. There are special assessment and monitoring charts that are filled in every hour by the ward nurses. These charts check the dose of medicine that your child is receiving and how effective it is. As your child's pain decreases the medicine is decreased as well.

CAN MORPHINE FOR PAIN CONTROL CAUSE ADDICTION?

Your child will not become addicted to the morphine that they are receiving as pain control. Addiction does not occur even if a child needs morphine for an extended length of time.

WILL MY CHILD EXPERIENCE UNPLEASANT SIDE EFFECTS FROM MORPHINE?

Sometimes morphine may make your child feel slightly sick or itchy. These side effects can be reduced by:

Adjusting the dose of morphine
Giving other medicines to treat the side effects – such as anti-sickness medicine
Over sleepiness is rare and should not be confused with your child 'catching up' on sleep that he or she may have lost if they were very unwell prior to surgery.

WILL MY CHILD BE SORE WHEN MORPHINE IS STOPPED?

We often give regular doses of milder pain relief medicines such as paracetamol or diclofenac at the same time as morphine. These can be given as a tablet, syrup or suppository. They can help us to use less morphine and to wean the morphine more speedily. When morphine is stopped these milder drugs are being given in adequate amounts to keep pain well controlled.

Contact Clinical Nurse Specialist, Pain Relief: Page 2133/ext. 0449. *Any problems: Monday to Friday: 0830 1700*

Subcutaneous Morphine Infusion

(Please place completed chart in casenotes)

Name................................Unit No.............D.o.B...............Age.............Weight.............

Operation...Date.....................................

Morphine Concn. (1mg/kg in 20 mls 0.9% Saline)..

Rate from...........mls/hr to ....mls/hr

Any adjustments (specify type, reason and time made).....................................

Infusion site: Deltoid Pectoral Abdominal

Serial No. of Pump..................................

Signature of Anaesthetist............................

Date & time commenced...............................

Record hourly

Time	SpO$_2$	Resp Rate	Sedation Score Eyes open: 0 = Spontaneously 1 = To speech 2 = To shake **3 = Unrousable (Call Doctor)**	Pain Score 0 = No pain A = Asleep 1 = Not really sore 2 = Quite sore **3 = Very sore (Crying)**	Nausea Score 0 = None 1 = Nausea only 2 = Vomiting x1 in last hour **3 = Vomiting >1 in last hour**	Rate of infusion (mls/hr)	Volume left in syringe

3 = Unrousable (Call Doctor)	2 = Quite sore 3 = Very sore (Crying) (Call Doctor)	>1in last hour (Call Doctor)	(not easily calmed) 3 = Severe inconsolable may need top up sedation (call Doctor)

CALL DOCTOR if pain score 3, nausea score 3; restlessness score 3;Syringe empty
CONTACT DOCTOR AND SWITCH OFF EPIDURAL if patient unrousable (score 3);SpO_2 <90%
block height above [ ] ; HR< [ ] ;BP< [ ]
CONTACT duty anaesthetist bleep 2602 if help needed, or Dr...Home no.................

Contact Clinical Nurse Specialist, Pain Relief: Page 2133/ext. 0449. Any problems: Monday to Friday: 0830 1700

Intravenous Morphine Infusion

(Please place completed chart in casenotes)

Name..Unit No....................D.o.B....................Age....................Weight....................

Operation..Date....................

Morphine Concn. (1mg/kg in 50 mls 0.9% Saline)..(maximum 50mg in 50mls)

Rate from............mls/hr to ....mls/hr

Any adjustments (specify type, reason and time made)..

Serial No. of Pump....................

Signature of Anaesthetist....................

Date & time commenced....................

Record hourly

Time	SpO$_2$	Resp Rate	Sedation Score Eyes open: 0 = Spontaneously 1 = To speech 2 = To shake **3 = Unrousable (Call Doctor)**	Pain Score 0 = No pain A = Asleep 1 = Not really sore 2 = Quite sore **3 = Very sore (Crying) (Call Doctor)**	Nausea Score 0 = None 1 = Nausea only 2 = Vomiting x1 in last hour **3 = Vomiting >1 in last hour (Call Doctor)**	Rate of infusion (mls/hr)	Volume left in syringe

268

CALL DOCTOR if severe pain (score 3), patient unrousable (sedation score 3), SpO$_2$ <90. Respiration rate less than 10 if over 5 years, less than 20 if under 5 years, excessive nausea or vomiting, drip blocked/tissued or pump alarming. If patient unrousable, switch pump off and consider naloxone, 10 micrograms/kg IV

CONTACT duty anaesthetist bleep 2602 if help needed, or Dr...Home no....................

Bupivacaine Wound Perfusion

(Please place completed chart in casenotes)

Name.................................Unit No.............D.o.B................Age.............Weight............

Operation...Date.................................

Bupivacaine Concentration: 0.125%   0.25%   0.375%   0.5%

Rate from............mls/hr to ....mls/hr

Any adjustments (specify type, reason and time made).................................

Infusion site:

Serial No. of Pump.................................

Signature of Anaesthetist.................................

Date & time commenced.................................

Record hourly

Time	SpO$_2$	Resp Rate	Sedation Score Eyes open: 0 = Spontaneously 1 = To speech 2 = To shake **3 = Unrousable (Call Doctor)**	Pain Score 0 = No pain A = Asleep 1 = Not really sore 2 = Quite sore **3 = Very sore (Crying) (Call Doctor)**	Nausea Score 0 = None 1 = Nausea only 2 = Vomiting ×1 in last hour **3 = Vomiting >1 in last hour (Call Doctor)**	Rate (mls/hr)	Volume left in syringe	Check site

CALL DOCTOR if severe pain (score 3), patient unrousable (sedation score 3), SpO$_2$ <90. Respiration rate less than 10 if over 5 years, less than 20 if under 5 years, excessive nausea or vomiting, or pump alarming.

CONTACT duty anaesthetist bleep 2602 if help needed, or Dr...................................Home no.............................
or   Susan Fisher   bleep 2133